HEALING, ONE
BRUSHSTROKE
AT A TIME

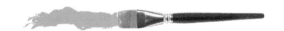

EXPRESSIONS OF BETRAYAL AND BEAUTY

Healing One Brushstroke At A Time, is a powerful resource and priceless gift for women bearing wounds of betrayal trauma. With intimate glimpses into the heartbreak and hope of her own unexpected journey, Sheila Paige blends vivid prose with her own soul stirring paintings through which she unexpectedly processed her own trauma. Without once settling for superficial religious remedies, she invites readers to know a God who knows us, welcomes us, and holds us—especially when everything is imploding. This book will be our new go-to resource for women in need of a wise and trustworthy guide through betrayal trauma.

MICHAEL JOHN CUSICK
CEO & Founder at Restoring the Soul, Author, Surfing for God: Discovering the Divine Desire Beneath Sexual Struggle

I absolutely LOVE this book! For years I've encouraged women to draw or paint if they can't find a way to release their painful emotions, but I lacked a resource specifically for partners of sex addicts to encourage them to use. But going forward, this book is my go-to resource for hurting partners whose painful emotions won't metabolize in other ways. And best of all, one doesn't need to have artistic technique or talent to portray their painful emotions in powerful ways that unlock and emancipate them from the cell of misery. They now have a jailer's key! Thank you, Sheila!

MARSHA MEANS
Marsha is the founder and director of A Circle of Joy Ministries. She trained as a Marriage and Family Therapist, and now works as a betrayal trauma coach. She is an author and also speaks on the topic of betrayal trauma and sex addiction. Marsha was at the forefront of a movement within the therapeutic community to understand sex addiction—infidelity, pornography, and other forms of sexually acting out—as causing a particular type of betrayal that traumatizes the addict's partner.

Pain, grief, wounds, shame, trauma, addiction, loss. These are only a few words to describe what a wife experiences when faced with sexual betrayal by her husband. Sometimes these words don't even come close to portraying the depth or breadth of such emotions. And that is where this book is beautifully unique. Sheila does a masterful job using both her words and her art to deliver a message of truth and grace and hope to women who are facing terrible heartbreak.

Healing One Brushstroke at a Time is a must read for any woman who has wondered if she will ever 'breathe' again. In this book you will discover a new vision for your life, even as you travel through your pain. A new life that includes such words as hope, faith, forgiveness, redemption, beauty, grace, and love.

JONATHAN DAUGHERTY,
Jonathan is the founder and director of Be Broken Ministries, and founder of Gateway to Freedom workshop for men. Jonathan also hosts the weekly radio broadcast, Pure Sex Radio, and is in demand nationally as a speaker on sexual purity and men's issues. He has appeared on The Oprah Show, twice on ABC's Nightline, as well as other radio and television media, both local and national. He has authored Grace-Based Recovery, The 4 Pillars of Purity, Secrets, Untangled and other works.

In this beautiful work, Sheila shares honestly about her journey through loss, pain and betrayal. Her experience is authentic, her words are healing, and her paintings are moving! If you find yourself in a place where you are struggling under the weight of wounds or trauma, I highly recommend this book. I believe that Sheila's story will give you greater courage for the story God the Father is writing in your life. Let her words inspire you, and they did me, as you read and absorb this work.

At the same time, I encourage all husbands and husbands-to-be to read this book! Sheila's words and personal story will remind you of what's at stake- what you're fighting for- on your own journey of purity. Her authentic experience will call you to a vision of godly manhood that could become a strong shield of integrity in your own marriage.

NICK STUMBO
Executive Director, Pure Desire Ministries,
Troutdale, Oregon
Author of Setting Us Free and Safe: Creating a
Climate of Grace in a Culture of Shame

What Readers are Saying About
HEALING, ONE
BRUSHSTROKE AT A TIME

ISBN Paperback: 979-8-9863972-0-7
ISBN Hardback: 979-8-9863972-2-1
ISBN eBook: 979-8-9863972-1-4

To all the brave women
who have shared
their stories.
Your honesty in
your pain is helping
me find a way
through mine.

Dear Reader,

I have thought about you and prayed for you as I have put words to my story.

For those of you reading this because you faced—or are facing—a similar path of betrayal trauma, my heart has ached for you. My eyes have welled up in tears for you. Nothing about this journey is easy. I pray this book will help you to feel seen and heard.

> It is my hope that it will be like first responders have arrived on the scene where you are lying, bloody and wounded.

> May you feel like your pain has been assessed and validated.

> May you receive CPR and life-giving oxygen so you can begin breathing again.

> May healing balm be applied to your wounds and may bandages keep you from bleeding out.

> May these words be the ambulance that takes you to places where you can receive more help and healing.

For those of you who may be reading this as the spouse who is struggling with sexual brokenness issues, may you be protected from condemnation as you read these words. My words were not written to heap more shame upon you. Even as you read of some of the pain that inappropriate sexual compulsions and acting out can bring, I hope you will know that the grace of God is deeper than any shame you feel. There can be hope, healing, freedom and recovery for you. I pray this book will lead you to resources that will help you in your own journey, even as the words bring you greater empathy for your spouse.

To pastors and ministry leaders, I'm sure you are already aware that the digital era we live in has greatly increased the availability and severity of pornography. The statistics are alarming concerning the numbers of people watching porn, and the numbers do not change whether or not the individuals are attending church. This means there are many under your leadership who are viewing pornography. Pornography is just one way that individuals are looking for affirmation, love, self-soothing and sex outside of the covenant of their marriage.

I hope this book will help you know how to begin walking with those hurting due to sexual brokenness. I pray you will address these complex issues and come alongside any in your flock struggling with sexual sin. There are many ministries that are willing to partner with you to help those who struggle with mental health and/or sexual integrity issues discover freedom and healing. I also hope this book will help you listen to betrayed spouses, respond to their deep pain, and give them the support that they need. They need to be believed and validated.

For family members and friends of those walking these hard roads, I hope this book will offer you some clarity and insight. I pray that you will become prayer warriors, truth-tellers and cheerleaders for those who are desperate for support and encouragement.

May each brushstroke (and key stroke) of this book be a message of God's love.

Sheila Paige

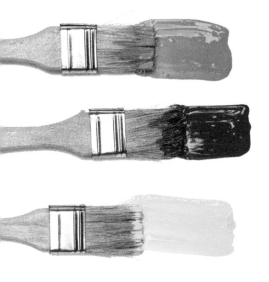

Contents

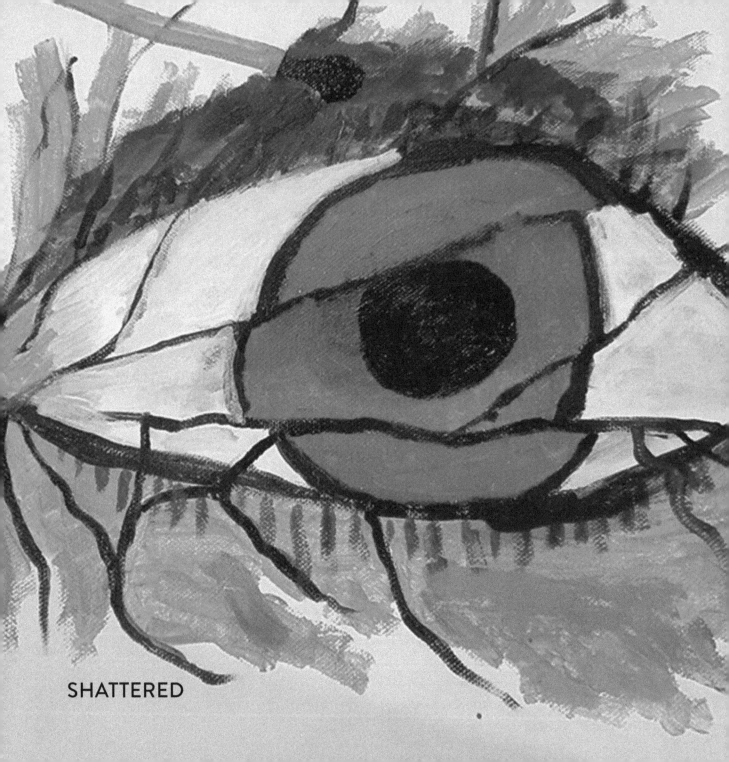

SHATTERED

1

Picking Up a Paintbrush

My soul is in deep anguish.
How long, Lord, how long?

(Psalm 6:3)

I'd lost the ability to write. How could I keep picking up my pen just to rewrite the same stories of pain?

How often could I record that I had been betrayed again? How could I find words to describe the cycle I was living in? Why try to put words to the tiny green shoots of hope I would begin to feel, only for them to inevitably be smashed in the dirt again?

At the beginning of 2020, I was at a crossroad. I knew that my husband was getting intensive treatment. At the end of these six weeks, if his mindset and the patterns of his compulsions had not changed, I knew I would need to make decisions I had not yet been able to face.

My world as a wife felt shattered. The repercussions of living in a world constantly shifting was affecting every area of my life.

I was exhausted after I had spent the last four and a half years since D-Day trying to find something that would help my husband and, in turn, help our marriage. In the betrayal trauma context, D-Day refers to Discovery Day or Disclosure Day. On that day your world is rocked, not only because of learning about sexual acting-out behaviors that had taken place that violated your marriage covenant, but also finding out that your spouse has worked hard to keep a part of his life hidden from you.

After D-Day, I plunged into a world of trying to make sense of the situation. The books had been read, the podcasts listened to, and the online courses completed. There had been multiple conversations with therapists, counselors, psychologists, psychiatrists, coaches, and mentors.

Yet, the patterns continued.

By this time, I was emotionally depleted.

I had heard that art therapy was supposed to be helpful in expressing emotions, and since I found myself unable to write, I decided to give painting a try. As a fifty-two-year-old who was not artistic in the least, I had little hope for it being helpful.

But I bought a canvas, one paintbrush, and a few small tubes of acrylic paint. I watched a YouTube tutorial of a lovely landscape and I tried to follow along with the instructions.

My piece looked nothing like the beautiful painting on the screen. I went to bed feeling even more like a failure.

The next day after work, I tried again. The results were the same.

So much for art therapy.

Three strikes and I would be done with this experiment. That night, instead of following a YouTube artist, I just focused on painting the colors and swirls of the emotions I was feeling. Eventually, I painted one eye on the canvas.

As I painted, something shifted in my soul.

A little bit of healing took place.

My painting sojourn had begun.

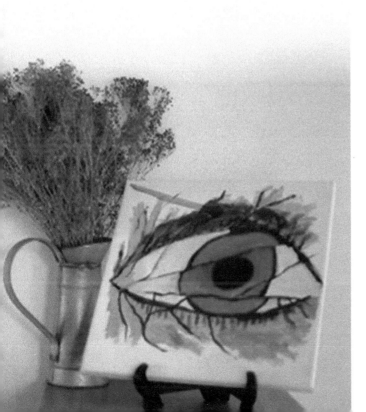

Questions *to* Consider:

1 If trauma has shattered the world you once knew, have any of the outlets below (or anything else) brought you some relief?

- plants, gardening
- your dog, cat, or other animals
- journaling or writing
- painting, drawing, pottery, photography or other artistic outlet
- walking, running, or other physical activity
- telling a trusted friend, counselor, coach or therapist

2 How has it helped?

3 Is there something new that you might want to try to help you on your healing journey?

4 What are some steps you could take towards making this happen?

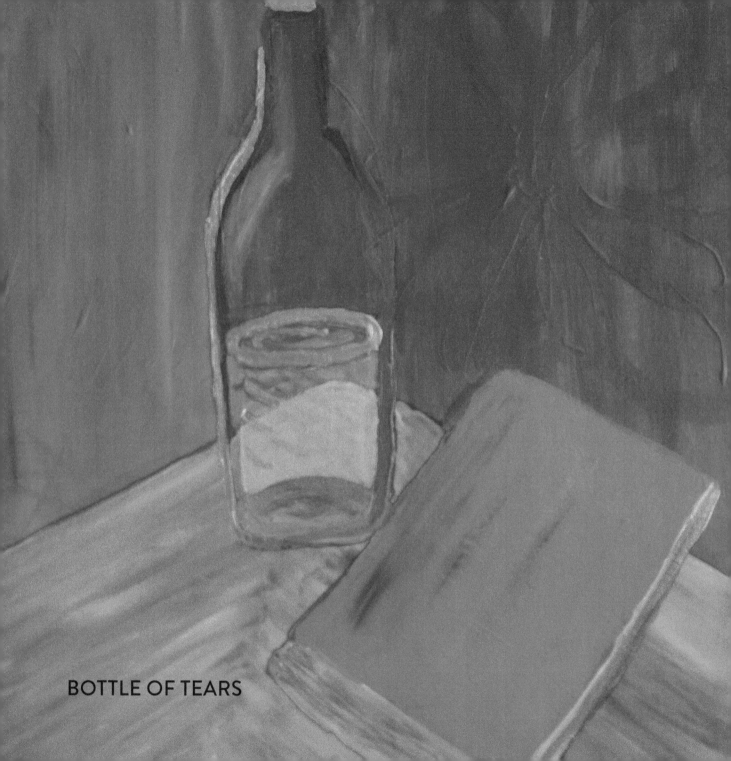

BOTTLE OF TEARS

2

Permission
to Be Sad

You keep track of all my sorrows.
You have collected all my tears in your bottle.
You have recorded each one in your book.

(Psalm 56:8 NLT)

The bottle for my tears must be a very large bottle.

With each revelation there was so much grief. So many losses.

'It wasn't supposed to be this way,' was the thought that seemed to go constantly through my mind.

It's natural to feel such a depth of pain when the dreams we've held since childhood come crashing down.

The prince is no longer pursuing the princess. In fact, his thoughts and fantasies are elsewhere.

The marriage you thought you had is not what you thought it was.

In my case, the grief I felt on D-Day was compounded again and again by new revelations. Just when I thought life was beginning to feel stable, another earthquake would occur. The truth-trickling kept me feeling off-balanced. The next shock wave brought all the pain and grief back again.

Raised in a Christian culture, an inaccurate message I subconsciously picked up was that as a Christ-follower, I needed to continually choose happiness. Even some songs I was taught from an early age reinforced this message:

Happy All the Time

I'm inright, outright, upright, downright
Happy all the time
Since Jesus Christ came in
And cleansed my heart from sin
I'm inright, outright, upright, downright
Happy all the time

Open Up Your Heart (And Let the Sunshine in)

So let the sun shine in, face it with a grin.
Smilers never lose and frowners never win.
So let the sun shine in, face it with a grin
Open up your heart and let the sun shine in.

When you are unhappy, the devil wears a grin

But oh, he starts a-running when the light comes pouring in
I know he'll be unhappy 'cause I'll never wear a frown
Maybe if we keep on smiling he'll get tired of hanging 'round.

I believed Jesus had died to save me from my sins and He had given me life. I was grateful for that. I don't know how I would have navigated through this great pain without my faith.

But, I discovered it was impossible to feel happy when my world had imploded. How can you choose joy when your heart is in a million pieces?

One unusual aspect of the betrayal journey is that you instinctively want to turn to your spouse for comfort. However, the very one you want to turn to is the one who keeps hurting you. It's so ironic that when I was in the most pain, I would long to be held by my husband because I loved him.

I had to learn to process my sad feelings in a new way.

During this journey, I've had to befriend Christ, the Man of Sorrows. One who had also been betrayed. I've discovered the necessity of lament. I've had to learn to become comfortable with sadness as an ever-present companion.

My betrayal trauma journey became a school of grief. I've learned I don't have to deny it or pretend it away.

There are legitimate reasons my heart feels shattered. It is okay to not be okay.

Each tear is a testament to my losses.

And God is okay with that. In fact, He has been tenderly collecting and keeping track of each one.

Questions *to* Consider:

1 What experiences in your past shape how you view sadness?

2 Have you been able to admit and lament over the grief and trauma in your life?

3 Have you ever had someone validate your pain and grieve with you? How did this feel?

4 At this moment in your life, do you believe that God cares about your sorrows? Why or why not?

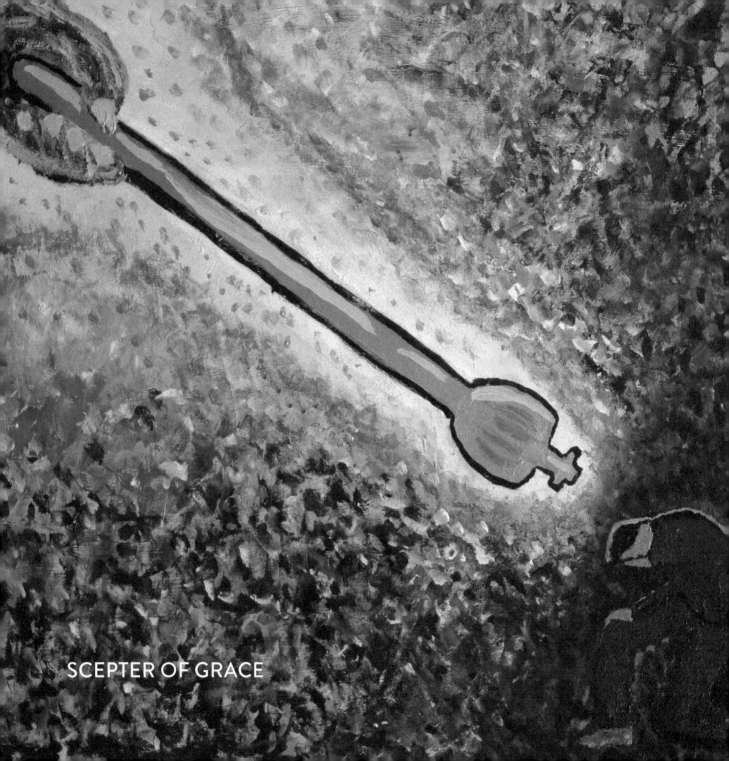

SCEPTER OF GRACE

3

Giving up
Control

When he saw Queen Esther standing
in the court, he was pleased with her and
held out to her the gold scepter that was
in his hand. So Esther approached and
touched the tip of the scepter.

(Esther 5:2)

After two months of not seeing each other, it was time for my husband to arrive home. It was the longest we had been away from each other since falling in love thirty-three years before.

I was hopeful. Surely this would be the turning point.

I was also scared. What if it wasn't?

When he arrived, it was so good to be in his arms again. To converse with someone across the table. To have a shoulder to lean on as we watched a movie. To share stories and catch up about our children. To once again look into the eyes of the person I had loved for so many years.

I had a million questions about his time away, but I tried not to overwhelm him. Through counseling, I had learned that this was something I often did that was hard for him. Since my mind processed quickly, I often threw too many questions or too much information at him. Knowing he was jet-lagged and tired, I tried to just enjoy his presence.

I did ask a few questions about a friend's prayer ministry he had attended on his way home. The husband and wife team had prayed over him. As I asked him about it, he showed me the paper where they had written down things that had come to their minds as they had prayed for him.

I read the words "a golden rod" and wondered what it might mean. I looked it up and discovered the story in the Bible about Queen Esther. I wondered if the golden rod might represent the golden scepter the King offered to Queen Esther. When she entered the King's presence, her life was in his hands.

When he extended his golden scepter to her, he offered her life. When she reached out and touched it, she accepted life.

Less than two weeks after arriving back home, my husband decided that living with me was just too hard. He said I was too controlling and that he needed space. He packed his bags and left.

I was left with a broken heart and some very hard decisions to make.

The image that kept coming to mind was that golden scepter being offered to my husband. Just as Queen Esther had the choice to receive the life it offered, I was aware we each have that choice as God offers the scepter of grace to us. I could reach up and touch it for myself, but I couldn't force my husband to make the life-giving decisions I wanted him to make.

As this image came to mind, I painted it, weeping. I so wanted to paint my husband's arm up, receiving the healing being offered to him. But that was not my role. It was time to stop fighting for his health and our marriage.

Letting him go was the hardest thing I have ever done.

As I had immersed myself in the recovery world since D-Day, I had heard these words time and time again: "You didn't cause it, you can't control it and you cannot cure it."

It was true. After four and a half years of fighting for his healing, it was time to let go.

It was no longer time to attempt to find the book or podcast or testimony or counselor or recovery plan that might make a difference. It was time to take my hands off of his life. To free him to make the choices he wanted to make.

So I painted and cried and released.

Questions *to* Consider:

1 If you picture God, the King of Kings, extending a scepter towards you, are you willing to reach up and accept the life He is offering you? Why or why not?

2 As you look at this painting, is there someone you love that you can imagine in the picture? Since you are unable to make their arm reach up and touch the scepter, what do you think your role is at this point in time...talking to them, sharing resources with them, praying for them, or releasing them? Something else?

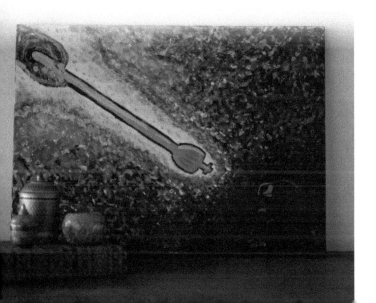

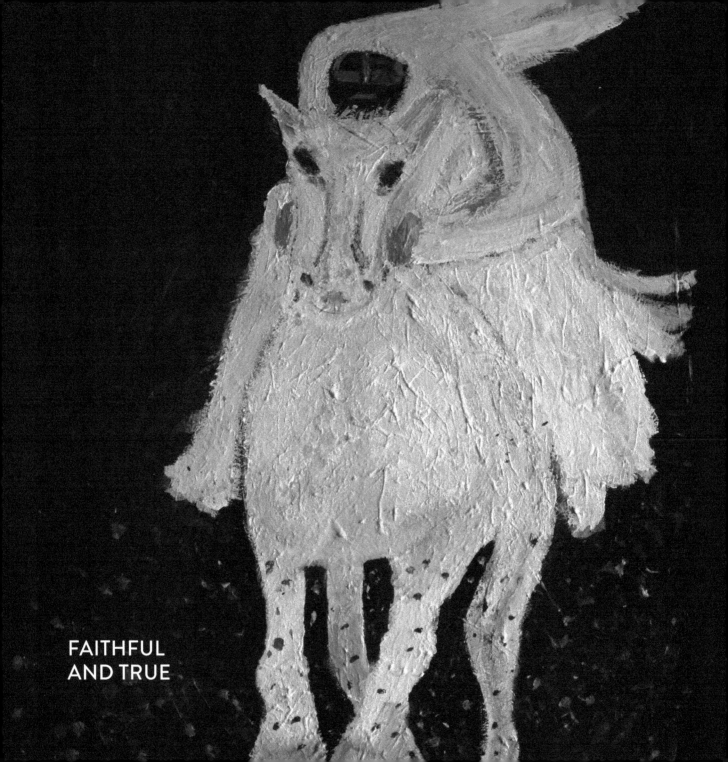

FAITHFUL
AND TRUE

4

In Need of a Rescuer

I saw heaven standing open and there
before me was a white horse, whose ruler
is called Faithful and True. With justice
he judges and wages war.

(Revelation 19:11)

I have two pictures of our dating years that stand out to me as confirmation that I was to marry this man. Several months after we began dating, we were driving through streets in a large strange city in two different cars. I was following the Volkswagen Bug he was driving. These were the days before cell phones, so I had to keep a close watch where he was going as we wound our way through all the red lights, traffic, and unfamiliar streets. As I gripped the steering wheel tightly and kept my focus on the blue "Herbie" car in front of me, I had the clear thought this was a picture of my life ahead and that I would be willing to follow the young man ahead of me wherever he would go.

Another night, we were on a ridge overlooking the city lights beneath us. It should have been a romantic evening, but we were at a point in our relationship where things seemed hard. We were having a difficult discussion about our relationship and if we were supposed to be together, and why it was sometimes hard. As I sat on the hood of my car crying, I looked down and saw a bit of green coming up between the cracks in the pavement of the parking lot. I jumped down and picked them up. There were two pea pods that had broken through the hard asphalt to grow and flourish together. I took it as a sign that even though things were hard, we were supposed to be together. We would make it through this hard time, and God would take care of both of us.

I had no doubts on the day he asked me to marry him, or on the day we said "I do" on January 1st, 1990. Throughout our marriage, I believed that the differences in our personalities were for our good. I never imagined that our marriage wouldn't make it. Finding myself in this place was crushing.

During those first days of coming to grips with the fact that there was nothing left for me to do to save my marriage, I kept picturing an image that Dr. Sheri Keffer had mentioned in her book, Intimate Deception. Dr. Keffer tells a beautiful story about a woman and her healing story that included a verse about Jesus as the Faithful and True One.

I clung to that mental picture of Jesus coming, thundering hooves pounding as he rushed to my rescue. A horse at full gallop, overcoming all obstacles as Jesus rushed to pursue His beloved daughter that had been wounded.

I felt like I was a heap in the mud, barely visible. I was wounded emotionally from unfaithful and untruthful words and actions. Yet, Jesus saw me in the puddle.

He knew that young lady who, years before, had agreed to follow that man in the Volkswagen Bug. He knew I never had any idea of some of the places that my husband's brokenness would take him. God knew I never imagined that one of the pea pods would grow in a completely different direction.

The ruler named Faithful and True was on His way to minister to my mangled heart.

I painted this as I tried to capture the urgency of the Rescuer towards the one He loves. I knew I would not make it through this next season without Him.

Perhaps you find yourself in the mud today, not even able to help yourself. May you begin to hear the hoofbeats.

Questions *to* Consider:

1 Make a list of the wounds in your heart that need healing.

2 As you find yourself in a place of pain, how does it make you feel to think of a Rescuer coming to your aid?

3 If you have been a recipient of unfaithfulness and deceit, how do the words Faithful and True impact your heart?

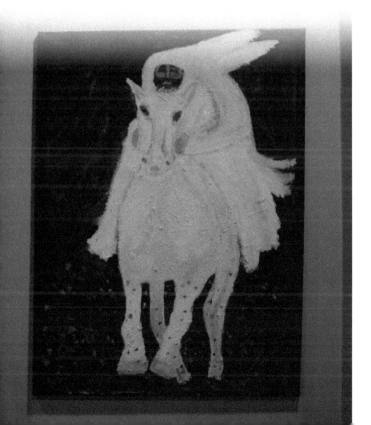

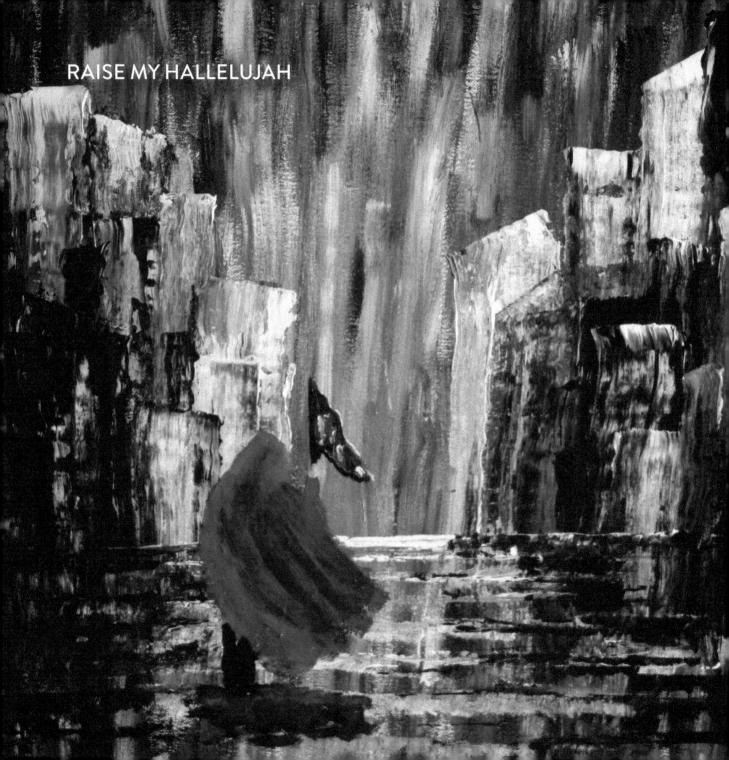
RAISE MY HALLELUJAH

5

Praise Him in the Storm

Though the fig tree does not bud
and there are no grapes on the vines,
though the olive crop fails
and the fields produce no food,
though there are no sheep in the pen
and no cattle in the stalls,
yet I will rejoice in the Lord,
I will be joyful in God my Savior.

(Habakkuk 3:17-19)

The first anniversary of my oldest son's death occurred just three months after my husband left. Not only was I re-living the phone call from the year before that rocked my world, but also, I kept thinking that my husband should be next to me, helping me to bear the weight of the day. Only the two of us had shared so intimately in the journey of our Kevin's life. Only the two of us would remember the stories and mourn his death as parents.

We had once been two young adults sharing God's love with those who lived in a housing project on the west side of Birmingham, Alabama. We had both fallen in love with Kevin, a little seven-year-old with a cowlick in the front of his hair and the friendliest brown eyes. We had poured love into him and let him live with us when his mother went to jail. Eventually, we adopted him.

We had loved Kevin through the years of ups and downs. The sweet and funny moments of his childhood. The turbulent teen years when he spent a lot of time in residential treatment. Our relationship with him had been restored when he was a young adult. We had loved him through his years in the army, and as he married and became a father to two sons.

We were devastated to find out that Kevin, at age 34, had gone into depression, and had taken his life. Suicide was never how we wanted our journey with him to end.

The storm inside me was raging.
The regrets.
The what-ifs.
The valley of the shadow of death.

Being without my husband in the agony only multiplied the pain. I was painting and crying while I listened to worship music. Then the song "Raise My Hallelujah" came on. Was it possible to raise my hallelujah on this day that marked broken dreams? Could I praise God after the pain of losing a son to suicide and in the midst of watching my marriage disintegrate?

I turned to YouTube to find some help with how to paint a storm. Then, I began to paint.

Finally, I painted myself into the picture.

A broken me, feebly raising a hallelujah in the middle of the storm. It was a tentative hallelujah that day.

A body weighed down by pain, barely able to raise an arm.

However, it was an acknowledgement that God was still good and worthy of praise. I knew that was true, even though I was swept up in a series of circumstances that were not good. Circumstances that had gutted my life.

Choosing to recognize God's goodness was an act of sacrifice for me that day. It was also one step forward on my healing journey.

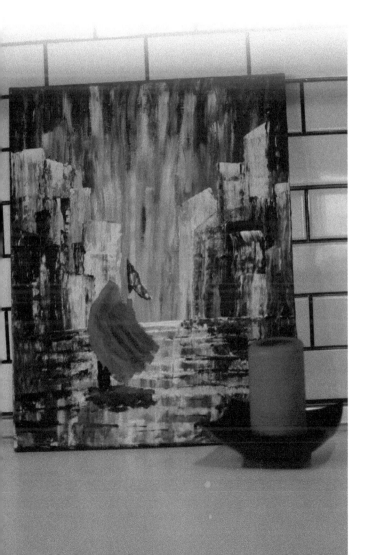

Questions *to* Consider:

1 Do you believe there is a God who is good and who cares for you?

2 Are you able to recognize His faithfulness and goodness even in the midst of your pain?

3 Are you able to "rejoice in the Lord" and "raise a hallelujah" during this time? Why or why not?

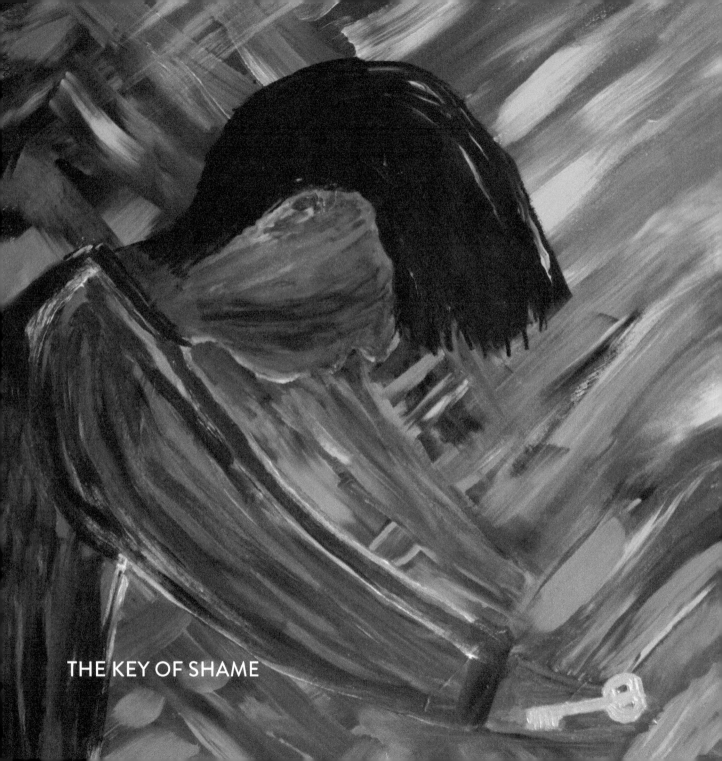

THE KEY OF SHAME

6

That Explains a Lot

When pride comes, then comes shame;
But with the humble is wisdom.

(Proverbs 11:2 NKJV)

One word kept coming up during counseling, and in the books and podcasts I was devouring. A word I had heard before but had never grasped how much power it had. The word shame. I knew the basic idea that when we did something wrong, we felt guilt and shame, but I never realized the power of shame and how much it impacts us. I never knew how shame could paralyze us and infuence our lives in countless ways.

I read a common way to differentiate guilt and shame is that guilt is the feeling you have when you know you have done something wrong. Shame is the feeling that you are bad.

Pride and shame are related. Pride drives us to look good in front of others, and as a result, shame pushes down unwanted issues and pretends that everything is okay.
It covers up.
It hides.

I can look back and recall many ways that shame influenced me. When a boy in my class in 6th grade called me gorilla because of my hairy arms, I became ashamed of my arms. Before that time, I wasn't even aware that my arms were hairier than normal (compared to my Dad's arms, mine were pretty smooth!)

When, as a third culture kid, I moved to the U.S. in 8th grade, I was proud of my pretty purple sundress that my Mom and I bought for Easter.

Until other teens asked where I bought my Easter dress. Apparently, K-Mart was not an acceptable answer and, because of shame, I learned how to divert answering questions about where I purchased clothes.

As a young teen, when I read passages in romances that revealed more about sex than I knew, shame kept me from telling anyone about it. I didn't know how, or feel safe enough, to share how the words made me feel—repelled, curious, and excited all at the same time.

As I studied sexual compulsions, brokenness, and addiction, I began to understand the reasons that someone would work hard to hide anything that didn't match up with the things they said they believed. It made sense that shame would prevent them from being honest about their desires and choices.

I realized that even my responses in the first twenty-five years of our marriage had most likely contributed to that feeling of shame in my husband. I had been shocked and appalled by some things he had shared with me, because I did not think Christian men should think those things. I can see how my reactions could send him into further hiding.

Since learning more about the role of shame in unwanted sexual behavior issues, I can see how the Christian church has failed to acknowledge sexuality and how that has led to increased shame in many Christians. I agree with psychologist Dr. Juli Slattery in her observations in her book Rethinking Sexuality: God's Design and Why it Matters, that we have failed as the Christian church to teach sexual discipleship. In ignoring the sexual brokenness that is part of who we all are, we have left our children and teens to be discipled by the culture around them instead. We haven't given Christian teens a safe place to talk about sexual curiosity.

I believe this is a key factor why so many Christians have porn addictions and other unwanted sexual behavior. They aren't able to share about their desires and choices, so it is kept hidden.

Unfortunately, shame generates an unhealthy cycle. When you feel unworthy, it can lead to you acting out in an inappropriate way to feel better about yourself. This shame inevitably generates more shame. Hiddenness is a key component in how addictions start and grow.

I've heard that shame spoken is shame broken, and I believe that is an important first step. Speaking out about our thoughts and activities is necessary to break habits that are hidden. Addictions begin with secrets.

I hope and pray we can become safe places for each other so we can begin to break the power of shame.

Questions *to* Consider:

1 Can you see ways that shame has impacted your own life?

2 In what ways do you think shame has impacted your loved one's life?

3 Does seeing the results of shame in your life and in the lives of others lead you towards more compassion towards others?

4 What illustrations or pictures come to your mind when you think of the impact of shame? Take a few minutes to sketch or write about the images that come to your mind.

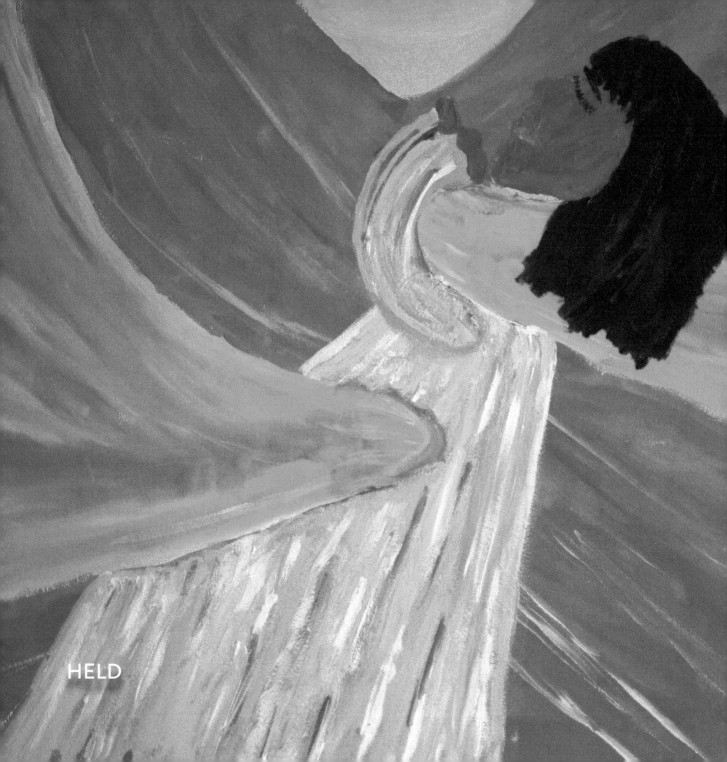

HELD

The Gift of My Body

Even my close friend, someone I trusted,
one who shared my bread, has turned against me.

(Psalm 41:9)

Between COVID restrictions and suddenly finding myself living alone after thirty years of marriage, I had been isolated, immersed in a deep well of grief. When a need came up in our community, I roused myself out of my cocoon to help out at a friend's house.

Her son had just been diagnosed with cancer, and she and her husband were spending time around the clock with their child at the hospital. They had five younger children at home. My heart ached that one day their lives had been normal, and the next, everything had been flipped upside down.

In some ways, I could relate.

They needed some extra bodies to help with their other children. I signed up for some night shifts when the children would be sleeping. One night when I was at their house, it was obvious the upheaval was taking its toll on them all. I finally got the younger children settled down. My friend came home from the hospital and spent time talking to me as she snuggled the baby. She was exhausted and made her way upstairs to sleep with her little one.

I stretched out on the couch, and later that night, I was awakened by a little girl who needed some comforting. I rocked her, sang to her, and eventually she fell asleep again. A little while later, her older sister appeared. She, too, needed some love. I wrapped my arms around her and rocked her to sleep.

Then, the Mom came downstairs with a very-awake baby girl. She handed her to me so she could return to get some sleep. I played with the bright-eyed little one. Eventually, her little body relaxed in my arms and fell asleep.

That night was so healing to me. I had gone weeks without any affectionate touch. Not only did I feel abandoned on a deep emotional level, but I also felt my body had been found wanting and had been rejected. On this night, three little girls needed me. They needed the comfort of my arms around them. They needed the safe place I could provide. They nestled their heads near my beating heart. Emotionally they needed love and care, but they also needed a physical body to hold them.

It was a moving, spiritual experience for me as God reminded me that my body was a gift. I often try to shove thoughts of my body away, yet it is part of who I am. God has given me my body, and it is valuable and needed.

As I held each girl, God reminded me He was holding me. I was not alone. I could almost feel His arms around me telling me I was loved during the chaos in my own life.

As soon as I got home, I tried to capture this feeling on canvas.

It speaks to me again and again.

I am valued.
I am loved.
I am held.

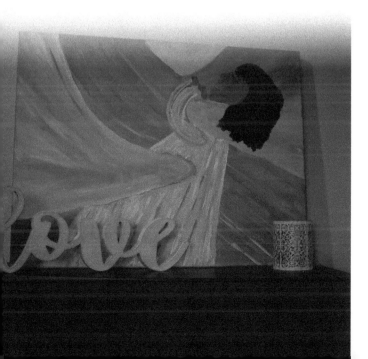

1 If someone you love has turned against you, which feelings below can you relate to?

- rejected
- betrayed
- unwanted
- undesirable
- insecure
- afraid
- others?

2 Have you had any experiences where God has reminded you you are loved and valued by Him?

3 Do you believe that your body is needed and valued by God? Do you believe that God sees you as beautiful and delights in you?

4 Can you imagine a God who holds you and sings over you? Take some time to sit with God, imagining being held close to His heart.

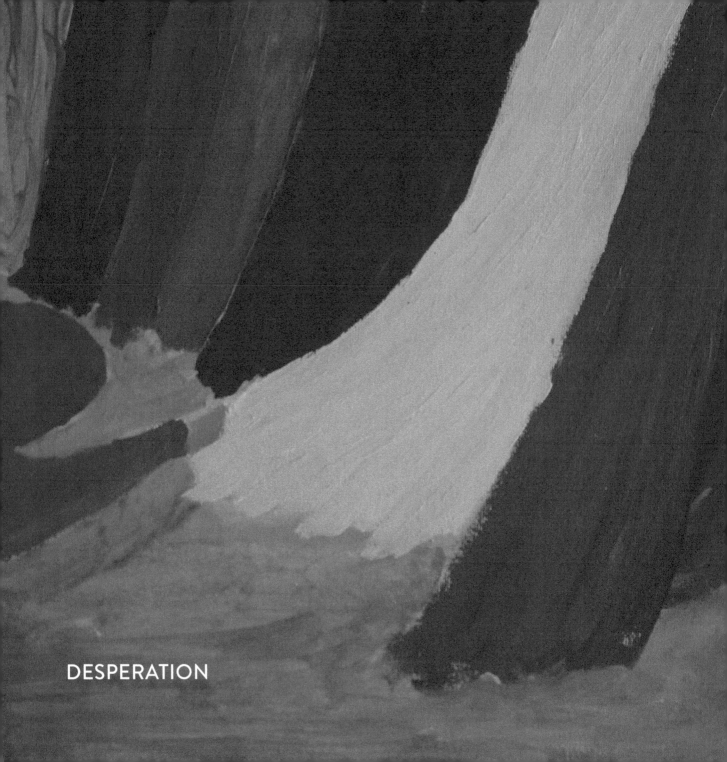

DESPERATION

8

Clutching
his Robe

A woman in the crowd had suffered for twelve years with constant bleeding. She had suffered a great deal from many doctors, and over the years she had spent everything she had to pay them, but she had gotten no better. In fact, she had gotten worse. She had heard about Jesus, so she came up behind him through the crowd and touched his robe. For she thought to herself, "If I can just touch his robe, I will be healed." Immediately the bleeding stopped, and she could feel in her body that she had been healed of her terrible condition. At once Jesus realized that power had gone out from him. He turned around in the crowd and asked, "Who touched my clothes?"

"You see the people crowding against you," his disciples answered, "and yet you can ask, 'Who touched me?'"

But Jesus kept looking around to see who had done it. Then the woman, knowing what had happened to her, came and fell at his feet and, trembling with fear, told him the whole truth. He said to her, "Daughter, your faith has healed you. Go in peace and be freed from your suffering."

(Mark 5:25-34)

The woman in the crowd didn't want to be seen, but her desire for healing drove her to seek a man with the reputation of a Healer. She didn't want to draw attention to herself. But, oh, how desperately she wanted healing after years of living with pain and shame.

I painted this while I was in a place of desperation.

How could the man I loved and trusted make decisions that hurt me time and time again?

How could I go on living as a missionary now that my husband had left me?

How could I explain what had happened and still honor the man I loved?

How could I face the world again when shame swirled in my head, telling me I was a failure because I was obviously not enough for my husband?

I was taking the first faltering steps towards legalizing the death of my marriage. The marriage that had been deeply injured with repeated confessions of broken marriage boundaries had taken the final breath the day he walked out.

In the book *Healing Your Marriage When Trust Is Broken: Finding Forgiveness and Restoration*, Cindy Beall quotes the words of a kind pastor that had made a difference to her. He said, "I would respect you if you felt that you needed to remove yourself from your marriage. What you've endured is very hard. But you are not a fool to stay and be a part of redemptive work in a man's life." I wanted to be a part of my husband's healing and redemption, too.

When D-Day occurred, I had taken a deep dive into learning all I could about why my husband may have made the choices he did and what could be done to help. As I learned about sex addiction, sexual compulsions, and intimacy anorexia, I was encouraged rather than discouraged. Over and over, I encountered stories of disclosure, hard work, restoration, and reconciliation. These stories were my lifeline, whether I was listening to the mentor stories in the Affair Recovery workshops or listening to stories on podcasts like Pirate Monk, Pure Desire, and Pure Sex Radio.

Even though I heard that it might take from eighteen months to two years to see real progress, I felt like that was doable. I wanted us to always be moving towards restoration. One of my children introduced us to the song "Broken Together" by Casting Crowns in the early days after D-Day. I took comfort in the lyrics that described a couple whose brokenness had caught up with them. As I listened to the message of shattered dreams and the desire to bring them to light in order to heal together, I longed for my husband and I to be broken together and to pursue healing together. But after years of trying, it was not headed in that direction.

This woman with the issue of blood became my friend during my dark and lonely nights. After putting her story on canvas, I hung it over my bed. At night, I would look up and see her hand clutching the robe of Jesus. I would reach out and clutch my sheet.

"Jesus, do you see me? I'm desperate, too. See me. Heal me."

In this story, Jesus doesn't just keep walking after the power in Him has healed the woman.

He stops.
He searches for her.
He validates her faith.
He heals her body and her heart.

For me there hasn't been instantaneous healing.
But I have often felt His presence with me.
Seeing me in my pain.
Assuring me I am not alone.
Tenderly calling me His daughter.
Reminding me that healing is possible.

Questions *to* Consider:

1 Have your emotions driven you to a place of desperation where you have tried to seek help in ways that have surprised you? Do you relate to any of the following?

- spending hours researching on the internet, trying to find solutions
- going forward at church to ask for prayer or asking to be prayed for at a Bible study, small group or prayer ministry
- talking to a mentor or pastor or counselor
- calling up a ministry you have only heard of on the internet
- joining an online group of like-minded sojourners
- going to a retreat on your own or asking your spouse to attend a retreat or going together
- paying money for an intensive or an internet program
- others

2 Do you feel a connection with this woman who fights through the crowds to touch the robe of the Healer?

3 Do you find yourself turning towards Jesus in your pain or away from Him?

4 What is your response when Jesus stops and turns to find her and then utters these words, "Daughter, your faith has healed you. Go in peace and be freed from suffering."

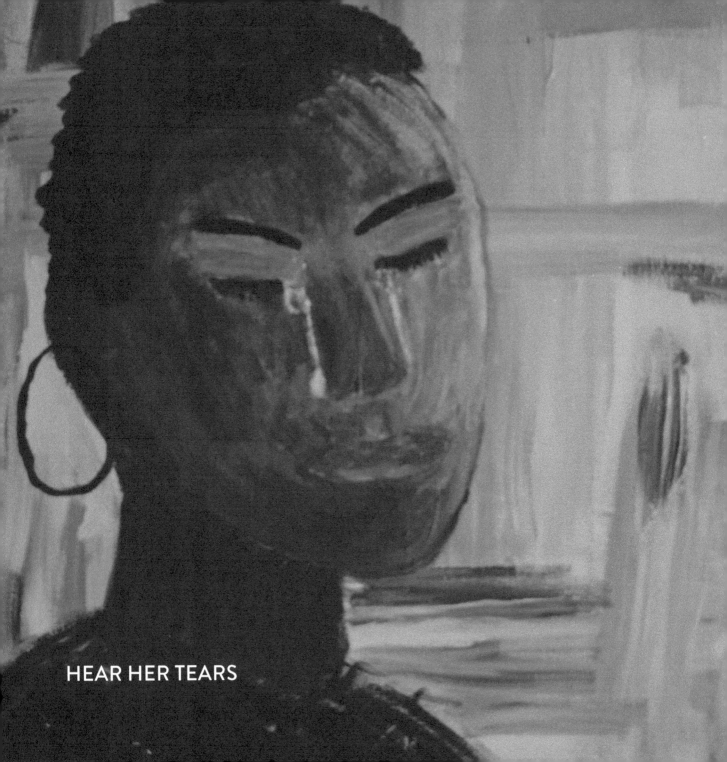

HEAR HER TEARS

9

The Impact of Trauma

The Lord is close to the brokenhearted and
saves those who are crushed in spirit.

(Psalm 34:18)

A lot of other hard things happened in the year 2020. A global pandemic resulted in the deaths of millions of people. Fear was escalating. International travel had screeched to a halt. Many of us were living in lockdown, unable to do the everyday things we took for granted. For those of us living across the globe from our families, we had no idea when we would see our loved ones in person again.

In addition, the killing of George Floyd brought to head the racial tensions in the U.S.A. Even though I lived in Thailand, the images of the trauma, anger, heartache, and chaos in the U.S.A. brought sadness to my heart. It had been less than a year since my own son's tragic death, and I felt empathy welling in me every time I heard of a mother losing her child to a senseless act.

The year 2020 was a year of trauma, not only for me personally, but also on a global scale. Before entering the betrayal trauma world five years earlier, I had given little thought to the word *trauma*. I associated the word with someone in a horrible car crash or a cruel beating. It wasn't until, trying to understand what was happening in my life, I took a deep dive into research and discovered the phrase *betrayal trauma* that I recognized that trauma put language to what I had been experiencing.

Trauma refers to extremely intense and distressing situations. When trauma occurs, our brain is overwhelmed to the point of not being able to regulate and process our emotions.

I learned that November 13, 2015 had been a traumatic event for me. I felt totally safe when I woke up that morning, sitting on the loveseat in our bedroom, praying and thinking about the day. My husband got up to go to the bathroom, and then came and sat next to me. I rested my head on his shoulder. I was happy and content. Our oldest daughter was flying to visit us in just a few days. I had no idea that the next words out of his mouth would be that he had something he needed to tell me. I also had no idea that it was to be the first of many, many conversations that would begin just like that.

The discovery that the person I loved and trusted had been keeping secrets pierced the world I knew. The continued truth-dripping and revelations caused accumulated trauma. Just like the majority of partners who experience betrayal trauma, my body was responding with Post-Traumatic Stress Disorder (PTSD.) That explained my racing heart, chest pain, stomach issues, panic attacks, and sleep issues. I also had emotional and mental symptoms such as anxiety, inability to concentrate, constantly feeling trembly, lightheadedness, and depression. I learned it was PTSD that made me jump anytime I heard a loud noise or sensed anything my body perceived as a threat.

I remember the days when I somehow made it through a work day, and my knees would buckle under me the minute I made it through the doorway of my home. I would collapse as the groans and tears came, finally being able to release the pent-up grief and sadness I had carried with me.

Understanding trauma helped me understand myself better and also gave me increased empathy towards others who have suffered. It made me wish I had understood trauma better when I had parented Kevin. He had endured so much trauma before we adopted him, and I now understood better why he had behaved the way he did. I am sad I never got to have a conversation about trauma with him.

It also gave me greater empathy towards my husband. Realizing that many men choose unwanted sexual behaviors to escape unresolved trauma from their childhoods helped me to have more compassion towards him. I realized that he had learned to turn to unwanted sexual behaviors as a way to self-soothe his own unregulated trauma.

One thing I have noticed in life is that people often tell us to "be strong" when we face a traumatic event. I know the intentions behind that are good. I believe it is said because others hope we will be strong enough to survive our grief.

However, it places pressure on the person going through the trauma. I don't think we can just decide to try harder and "pull ourselves up by the bootstraps" or white-knuckle our way to doing better.

When we have been traumatized, we don't need to try to "be strong." We need to heal. We need compassion. In Aundi Kolber's book *Try Softer: A Fresh Approach to Move us out of Anxiety, Stress, and Survival Mode–and Into a Life of Connection and Joy,* Aundi encourages her readers that rather than trying harder, we try softer.

I hope I will offer myself, and others, the softness of grace needed because of the trauma we have faced.

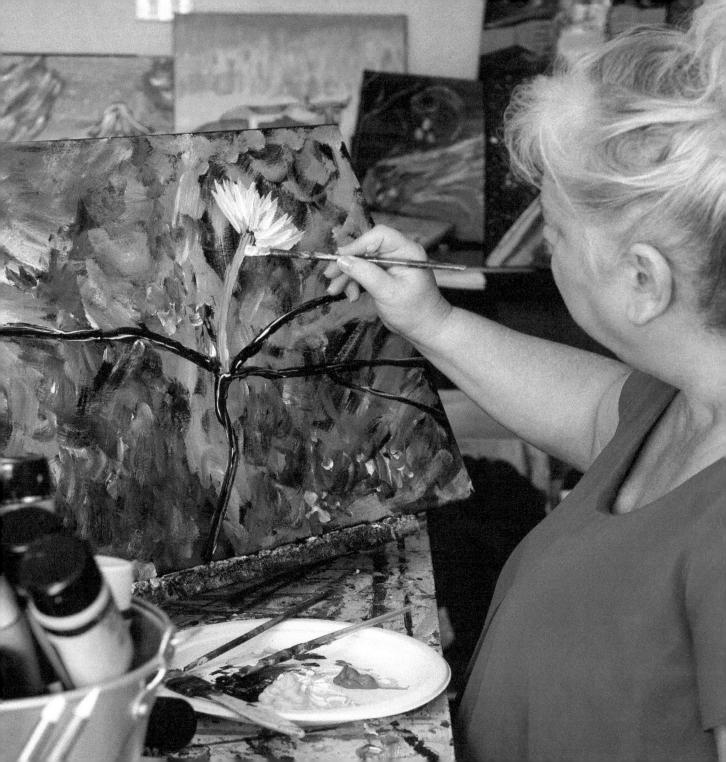

Questions *to* Consider:

1 Take a look at the following list. Have you observed any of these physical reactions that your body has experienced due to trauma?

- increase in heart rate
- fatigue, exhaustion
- feeling jumpy
- digestive issues
- headaches
- trembly, shaking hands
- others?

2 Can you discern any emotional symptoms that might be a result of trauma in your life?

- triggers, intrusive thoughts and flashbacks
- unable to concentrate
- confusion
- anxiety
- numbness
- sadness
- others?

3 Is your tendency to "white-knuckle" and to just try harder when you encounter hard things?

4 Can you think of some ways you could be gentler with yourself? How could you try "softer" rather than "harder"?

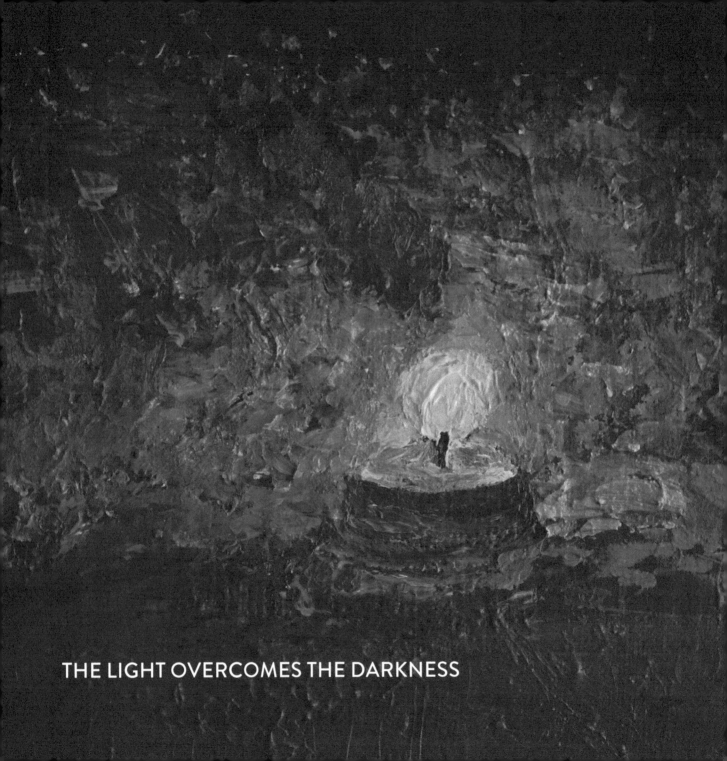

THE LIGHT OVERCOMES THE DARKNESS

The
Enemy

The thief comes only to steal and kill and
destroy; I have come that they may have life
and have it to the full.

(John 10:10)

The Lord your God is with you,
the Mighty Warrior who saves.
He will take great delight in you;
in his love he will no longer rebuke you,
but will rejoice over you with singing.

(Zephaniah 3:17)

When the person you trusted proves untrustworthy, it is natural to experience a huge amount of anger alongside your shock. During those first few days after D-Day, not only was I stunned and in agony, but I also was very angry. I don't apologize for that. It makes sense for someone to be angry when promises are broken.

However, during those first few days as I cried out in pain to God, I sensed Him revealing something to me that would make a difference during the next few years as I tried to understand my husband and fight for my marriage. I felt the Spirit of God whisper to me that my husband was not the enemy. He reminded me that the enemy was the "father of lies", the thief who sets out to steal and kill and destroy. This was a battle between Light and Darkness, not a battle between a wife and her husband.

Here is a poem I wrote based on Zephaniah 3:17. It was written for an online group of women who shared similar stories to mine.

Singing Warriors

We serve a God who is a Warrior who sings.
And, He enables us to be singing warriors.
Just as he fights for us, he has invited us to join Him in the battle.
And, the enemy is not our husbands.
The enemy is the one who has ensnared our husbands.

The one who has deceived them and blinded them.
The one who is out to steal, kill, and destroy.
The one who uses darkness and hiddenness.
Who tempts and then, when the deed is done,
Heaps on shame so that returning to God (and to us) feels unbearable.
We find ourselves here in this place.
In this battle that we didn't see coming.
That we didn't sign up for.
That has knocked us to the ground.
And often leaves us as a puddle on the floor.
But, again and again we rise up,
Slowly, hesitantly.
Inch by inch rising to take our place as warriors.
To fight against the enemy.
To fight for truth.
To fight for health.
We fight for our husbands.
As we do so, we are fighting for our marriages.
For our children.
For future generations.
But, even if the marriage is not restored.

We choose to pray.
We want to see every Christian man (and woman)
Walk free of sexual brokenness.
Walk free of hiddenness.
Walk free of broken vows.
Walk free of regret

God also invites us to sing.
To worship Him even as the all-too-familiar tears
Find their paths down our faces once again.
He invites us to cling to His goodness even in the midst of the storm.
He invites us to join Him in the song He sings over our husbands.
The song of redemption.
The song of forgiveness.
The song of resurrection.
The song that calls out the spark that God put inside our men—
That image of God that is there.
That always has the potential to choose...
Redemption,
Hatred of sin,
Recovery,
Restoration,
Empathy
Coming out of isolation and
Walking in community.
We join this song because of love.
Because even though we have been hurt more than we ever dreamed possible,
We also believe in the man we fell in love with.
We believe that he can be the man He was created to be.
We believe he can walk in honesty.
We believe he can resist temptation.
We believe he can learn to love.

We believe this because he is God's beloved, too.
We believe this because we know the God of the impossible.
We believe this because we believe in the power of the gospel.
Because we believe in both truth and grace.
However, if the man we love chooses to remain...
Remain in his lies
Remain in the darkness
Remain in his pattern of giving in to temptation
Remain in choosing death over life...

We will still know that we have a Singing Warrior
Who delights in us and who saves us.
We know no matter what happens
We are loved by the One who knows us best
By the One who weeps when we weep
And by the One who understands betrayal all too well.

Questions *to* Consider:

1 How does shifting the status of "enemy" from a human who has betrayed or abused you to Satan, the father of lies, make a difference in the way you think about your reality?

2 What is your response to the idea that you have a Singing Warrior singing over you and fighting for you?

3 How does the image of light overcoming the darkness speak to you?

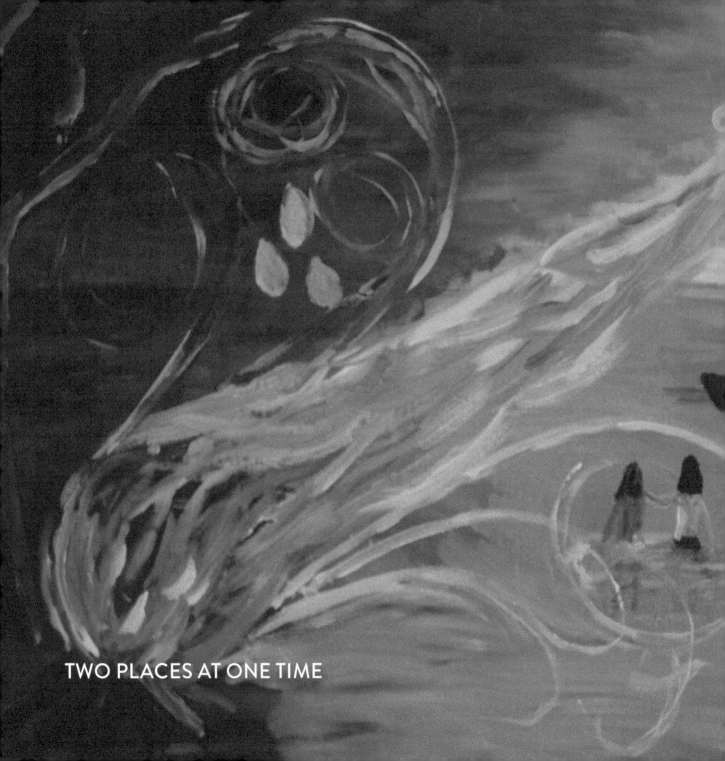

TWO PLACES AT ONE TIME

11

Triggered

When they landed, they saw a fire of burning coals there with fish on it, and some bread. Jesus said to them, "Bring some of the fish you have just caught." So Simon Peter climbed back into the boat and dragged the net ashore. It was full of large fish, 153, but even with so many the net was not torn. Jesus said to them, "Come and have breakfast." None of the disciples dared ask him, "Who are you?" They knew it was the Lord. Jesus came, took the bread and gave it to them, and did the same with the fish.

(John 21:9-13)

With one smell, we can be transported.

Or, maybe it is a sound
a location
a song or
a picture.

When you have experienced multiple traumas, it seems like every day is a minefield of triggers.

There are the triggers of the happiest of memories. Only now, they bring up so many questions and grief.

"What was really going on in his mind that day? How could I be so oblivious? I am so stupid."
"I can never go back to being that carefree again."
"The family we had that I was so proud of and grateful for is now torn and fractured."
"I don't know if I can ever make those cookies again because they remind me of him."

Or, the triggers bring the hardest of memories.

The anniversary of D-Day.
Or waking up in the night and being reminded of how often confessions came at this hour.
The location that screams at me to remember the time his anger exploded when we were standing right there.
Or I see something or read something that brings back a message that punched me in the stomach.

Suddenly, I am transported in time.

I'm reminded of Peter when I think about being in two places at the same time. He was triggered when he heard the rooster crow while he was standing at a fire warming his hands. He knew he had done exactly what Jesus had predicted. Was he triggered again, after the resurrection, when Peter smelled the smoke as Jesus cooked breakfast on the shore? Was he taken back to the night when he denied Jesus? Was he immediately transported back to the feelings of fear, shame, regret, and sadness that marked that horrible night?

If so, how amazing that Jesus used a fire again to display his love for Peter.

Jesus not only fed Peter's physical body that morning, but he nurtured his soul as well.

Just as Peter had denied him three times, Jesus now repeats a vision and purpose to Peter three different times.

Jesus redeemed the triggered memory. He gave Peter the gift of a grace-filled present tense now. The past was in the past.

When my triggers come, and I spiral down into a place of hurt and grief and sadness, I ask God to remind me that

His story for me isn't over yet. I remind myself that I am living in a grace-filled present tense moment now. I acknowledge that I am having a sad memory, but also remind myself that it is in the past.

I know my triggers will never be entirely gone. My memory bank with my former husband can't be rivaled by any other relationship I have had— the two of us have spent more time together than with anyone else in our lives.

However, their power over me can be lessened as they become reminders of the God of redemption rather than a desolate place.

Questions *to* Consider:

1 What are some of your most common triggers?

2 What can you do to remind yourself that even triggers of trauma, sadness and shame can be redeemed?

3 Just as the disciples ate breakfast with Jesus on the beach, how can you spend time in communion with Him? Is there an image that comes to mind when you think about spending one-on-one time with God? Take some time to draw or write about what you picture.

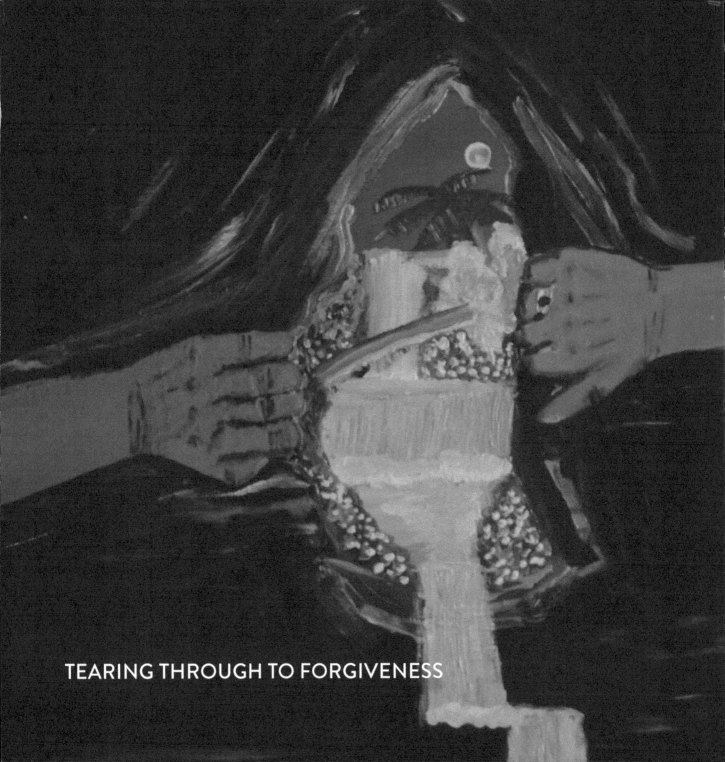

TEARING THROUGH TO FORGIVENESS

12

The Weight of Unforgiveness

Be kind and compassionate to one another,
forgiving each other, just as in Christ God
forgave you.

(Ephesians 4:32)

Some actions are hard to forgive.

Having my trust in my husband destroyed repeatedly was one of the hardest things about betrayal trauma. Studies show that spouses are more likely to be hurt more by the deception than the actual acting-out behaviors of the unfaithful spouse.

Addiction and mental health disorders are also often accompanied by impulsivity and sudden anger. This was a part of my former husband's story. As a result of this, I would find myself in uncomfortable and dangerous situations.

Watching my children hurt is also another arena that has caused me much pain on this journey, and whenever these hurts feel fresh and raw, anger pulses through me. I want my former spouse to experience some of the pain I am feeling.

Unforgiveness sits like a warm, inviting blanket over me. It feels like an appropriate place to feel the hot emotions that consume me. It makes my fingers race over the keyboard as I respond to another hurt. It's a place where I can let my wounds fester.

To be honest, I want to be trapped under that blanket for a while. I want to feel the anger throbbing through my body.

He deserves the angry thoughts I am feeling.

I have been so hurt.

It is not fair that I am experiencing broken promises once again.
I welcome the heat of anger in every cell of my body.

I'd rather feel the anger than the immense sadness that his actions bring to my heart.

I look at God's righteous anger against sin, and I know He also hates deceit. He hates seeing his beloved children being hurt. He had such great wrath against evil that it had to be poured out against the wrongdoers. It was fully poured on Jesus at the cross, and it was horrific. For a while, I can sit in that place and feel the wrath and injustice.

It feels good. Yet, eventually, it smothers me.

It's not healthy for me to stay in that raging and unforgiving place.

I need to also see another aspect of the Gospel. I need to hear Jesus on the cross saying, "Father, forgive them for they know not what they do." I need to hear Jesus explaining to Peter that forgiveness needs to occur repeatedly. Seventy times seven.

Every time I come to that crossroads of being faced with the choice to forgive or not forgive, I eventually need to get to the place to choose forgiveness again. It's an intentional choice I have to make to remove the heaviness off of me. To see beauty again, I will have to choose to grab hold of the blanket at some point and tear it apart.

It's usually not something that happens right away. Sometimes, the pain knocks me down and so far back that I can't even see that I have any options in the darkness. I have to acknowledge and process the pain first.

Eventually, though, I am faced with a choice.

It's a choice that God asks me to make because I, too, have been forgiven.
It's a choice that enables me to return to a place of love and compassion.
It brings me to a place where I can intercede for my former husband once again.

As long as the heavy blanket is encompassing me, I will never truly embrace the beauty of life again.

So, I forgive. I choose to rip the blanket off of me. I see beauty on the other side.

But then, I'm blindsided by a new discovery. Or, I find myself crying as I go through our pictures, his belongings, or our keepsakes. Or, I see my children's pain and it breaks my heart.

Once again, I'm faced with a choice.

Eventually, I choose to go through the process of forgiveness one more time. The beauty of my relationship with God and the absence of bitterness are worth it.

Questions *to* Consider:

1   How do you react when you hear the word 'forgiveness'?

2   If you look at forgiveness as a spectrum, which direction would you put your tendency–trying to push the pain down and forgive quickly without acknowledging the pain caused, or not granting forgiveness at all?

3   What do you feel God is speaking to you in this moment about forgiveness?

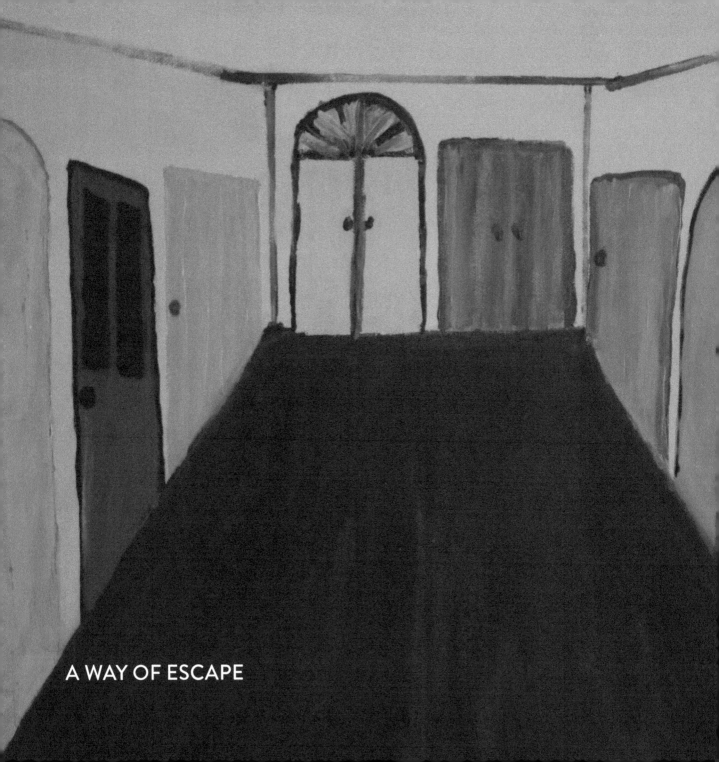

A WAY OF ESCAPE

13

Escape Room

No temptation has overtaken you except what is common to mankind. And God is faithful; he will not let you be tempted beyond what you can bear. But when you are tempted he will also provide a way out so that you can endure it.

(I Corinthians 10:13)

Part of the reason my story has been so complicated is the state of my former husband's mental health. Fifteen years into our marriage, he was diagnosed with OCD. Soon after D-Day, he was diagnosed with Bipolar Disorder. At the time of each of his diagnoses, we were thankful there was a reason and a name for some of the behaviors, intrusive thoughts, and psychotic thoughts. It also endeared him to me all the more, because I realized he was in a continual battle in his mind as he fought temptations he didn't want.

When he lost his job four months after D-Day, I was very sad for him. He had worked nineteen years in the same place and he was beloved in the community. It was hard to see it all come crashing down after one angry episode at his workplace.

It seemed like poor mental health narrowed down his thinking to where he could only see a limited number of options. Instead of seeing many possibilities of moving forward, he usually felt locked into just a couple of scenarios. Often, it was hard for me to know what was a mental health issue and what decisions were due to sin. Or, how much they overlapped.

Kathy Allen, working for Cornerstone Counseling Foundation in Chiang Mai, Thailand counseled my former husband and me for many years. She told us that although mental illness does contribute to many issues such as impulsivity, anger, and intrusive thoughts, it is not an excuse for sin. She reminded us often that God's Word includes a promise that there is always an escape from sin.

Escape oftentimes looks different than we may picture it.
We so often want it to be a dramatic rescue.
A billboard shining in the night.

Instead, it may mean picking up a phone to call a friend. It may mean checking in with someone every day. It could look like learning to give words to our emotions.

It was impossible to know how much mental health impacted my husband's sinful decisions. I wanted to be compassionate and understanding, but it was often difficult to know how to respond when my heart was breaking.

It's also hard to feel like you carry the weight of responsibility for a loved one's mental health. If you tell them that what they have done has hurt you, will it send them down a spiral of depression? If you explain how you feel, will they respond in an irrational and rage-filled way?

Living with the fear that something you say may cause suicidal actions is a heavy weight.

For me, it felt like I was always living on shaky ground. I never knew which step might send us into chaos.

Three years into my betrayal trauma journey, I was put on medication for anxiety and depression. The psychiatrist described it as "situational depression" because of the unsteady environment I lived in daily. For the first time I learned what it was like to live with thoughts that tormented me in a debilitating way.

I have spoken to many people who have loved ones who struggle with mental health. One friend recently shared with me that it is one topic she wants to talk to God about when she gets to heaven. It simply doesn't make sense to us why so many people go through so much torture and darkness in their thought life.

I ache for those struggling with mental health issues. I also ache for their loved ones, who often end up on a hard mental and emotional path as well.

When my husband was diagnosed with Bipolar Disorder, I remember reading that 90% of marriages with a partner with Bipolar Disorder will not survive. I was determined that we would beat the odds.

Unfortunately, it didn't happen that way.

For anyone struggling or has a spouse grappling with mental instability today, I encourage you to let a loved one or a professional know immediately. I do believe there is a way of escape out there, and I pray God will lead you to it.

Questions *to* Consider:

1 Have you or a loved one had to deal with mental health issues? If so, what has been the hardest part of that journey?

2 What would you ask God about mental health if you were sitting down with Him face-to-face today?

3 What has been helping you with your mental health throughout this stressful time?

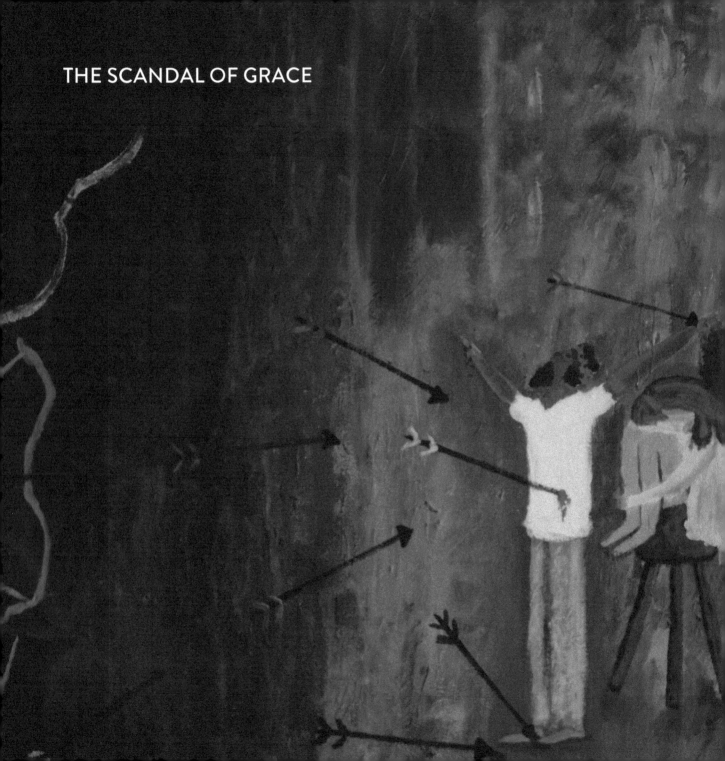

THE SCANDAL OF GRACE

Present Tense
Gospel

"He himself bore our sins" in his body
on the cross, so that we might die to sins
and live for righteousness; "by his wounds
you have been healed."

(I Peter 2:24)

There have been many songs that have helped me through these last few years. One of these is "Scandal of Grace." I love the emphasis it gives to what Jesus has done for us so that we may live. There were many nights I could not sleep and I would go out on my balcony and listen to this song on repeat.

When my wounds were raw and aching, I needed to go back to the gospel. I needed to cling to the good news that Jesus had already died in my place. When shame overwhelmed me, it was important to remember that it was through the wounds of Jesus that I was healed. When the knowledge and awareness of my own sin weighed my heart down in heaviness, I had to remember that Jesus died so that I wouldn't have to live with the weight of my sin.

In listening to the Pirate Monk podcast, I have often heard Nate Larkin share that we need to live in the present tense gospel. The gospel is not just about discovering God's love and admitting our sins once as we make a choice to become a Christian. It is about daily recognizing our current sin and daily acknowledging that Jesus has taken the punishment meant for us.

I realized that I had an inaccurate picture of walking with Christ. I thought success as a Christian was living a life that others could see and desire. A life of hope, happiness, and joy birthed in my decision to follow Christ and lived out by right choices. I thought it was important that my marriage and my family reflect a Christ-centered home. I hoped to bring that good example to Thailand.

I was learning that the only good example is Jesus. Just like the rest of the world, I couldn't get my life together in the way I wanted. The truth is that no one can. We are all imperfect beings living in an imperfect world.

I was learning that there was no such thing as a "good Christian." Instead, successfully walking with Christ looked more like one who cradles the gospel tightly to themselves in their brokenness, even as they extend it to others who are broken too.

A picture that came to mind often during my days of recovery was that of Jesus jumping in front of me to take the arrows of accusation, guilt, shame, and sin. When the Enemy sent an arrow to pierce my heart—perhaps to accuse me once again of unworthiness or to berate me for not handling things better, I could just see Jesus stepping in front of me. I could picture Him receiving the arrows in my place.

One arrow that most women (including me) struggle with during betrayal trauma is the thought that we aren't enough, and that it was our fault that our husband's eyes turned elsewhere. This arrow of accusation and blame comes from the father of lies, the enemy of our souls. This arrow is not true.

Unfaithfulness is a sinful choice made because of our husband's own unresolved issues. No matter what a spouse has done, the decision to go outside of the marriage boundaries for pleasure or comfort is a sinful choice. It is not the betrayed one's fault.

It's a deep wound, but what a comfort it is to know that because of the wounds that Jesus took on our behalf, we can be healed.

My part is to believe it is true.
To believe that He has taken the punishment for my sin.
To believe that He has taken the arrows of shame for me.
To have faith in something that I hope for, even when I do not have evidence of what I cannot see.

It's very good news.

Questions *to* Consider:

1 As you look at this image, can you name some of the arrows of sin and shame that have been sent to target your heart?

2 As you picture Jesus stepping in front of you to take those arrows in your place, how does that make you feel?

3 When you feel the arrows coming, how can you remind yourself that Jesus died on the cross so that you don't have to live a life of burdens, guilt and shame?

4 Is there a verse or an image you could place in a prominent place to remind you that you are forgiven and that it is by His wounds that you are healed?

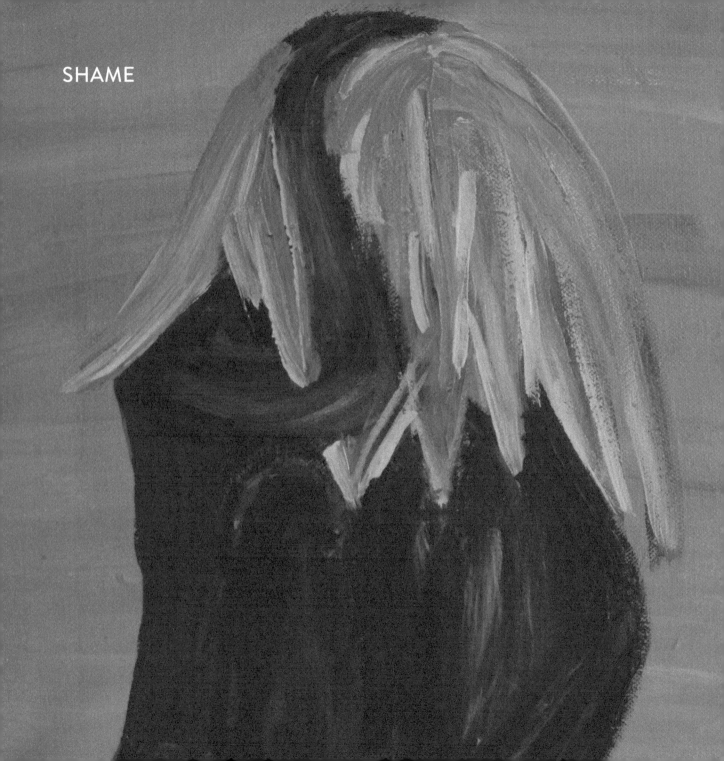

15

I'm Hiding
I'm Hiding

Where can I go from your Spirit?
Where can I flee from your presence?

If I go up to the heavens, you are there;
if I make my bed in the depths, you are there.

If I rise on the wings of the dawn,
if I settle on the far side of the sea,

even there your hand will guide me,
your right hand will hold me fast.

If I say, "Surely the darkness will hide me and
the light become night around me,"

even the darkness will not be dark to you;
the night will shine like the day,

for darkness is as light to you.

(Psalm 139:7-12)

But you, O Lord, are a shield about me,
my glory, and the lifter of my head.

(I Peter 2:24)

For me, going through both my son's suicide and the divorce left me wanting to hide. I wasn't ready to face the questions, and even the sympathy. I think one reason I wanted to hide was the sense of shame.

Suicide had been my son's choice for escaping from pain. My husband made unfaithful choices and chose to walk out on me. Yet, there still was the sense that I had done something wrong. There was still the feeling that I needed to hang my head.

I have learned there is a shared shame or social shame when we carry someone else's shame. Perhaps we feel like it is partly our fault. Maybe we are trying to protect them, so we can't tell others the truth about what happened. Maybe our own pride doesn't want us to admit the truth about how our lives have turned out.

And, of course, Satan, the father of lies, heaps more shame upon us.

'If you had been a better wife, your husband wouldn't have been tempted to look at others.'

'You are so hard to live with that your husband had to leave you.'

'If you had been a better mother, your son would have turned to you instead of taking his own life.'

'You are so undesirable that your husband had to leave you in order to find someone more attractive.'

Those accusations are hard. My personality type is one where I naturally think I have done something wrong and it must be my fault. So, I have had to work hard to replace the lies of shame with the truth that brings freedom. Even though I have the head knowledge that other people are responsible for their own choices, it is still hard for my heart to believe this. I have heard that the longest journey is the eighteen inches between our heads and our hearts. That resonates with me because I can know something and still have to wrestle to believe and rest in the truth.

I've discovered that desiring solitude is okay. I need time alone to withdraw from the crowds, to grieve, and to rest. Sorrow is exhausting.

There are also times when being alone is not healthy. When I withdraw and don't let others know that I am struggling and having a hard time with my grief and my thought life, I am isolating. When this happens, being alone is not good for me.

This is something I'm still trying to understand.

I'm trying to learn to read my heart on when I need alone time and when it will not be good for me.

Sometimes I feel like a turtle, poking my head out for a little while to see how I do around people and then retreating again.

Brene Brown, a well-known researcher and author defines shame as "The fear that something we have done or failed to do, something about who we are or where we come from, has made us unlovable and unworthy of connection." When I find myself withdrawing for this reason, it is important to connect with someone who is a truth-teller in my life. There are friends, family members and counselors who love me and can remind me that I am not unlovable or unworthy of connection.

When I was a little girl, my favorite poem was by Dorothy Aldis. The first stanza said, "I'm hiding, I'm hiding and no one knows where, for all they can see is my toes and my hair." It was a humorous take on the way toddlers think they are hiding, but they can still be seen.

That's how it is with God. Even when I want to hide, I can never hide from Him. I don't need to hang my head in His presence. He knows me fully and, yet, loves me completely.

Questions *to* Consider:

1. Do you feel a need to hide? Are you able to discern the difference between a healthy need for solitude and unhealthy isolation?

2. What drives you to want to hang your head?

3. Do you believe that God can be the Lifter of your head? Can you imagine yourself walking through life with your head lifted – not in a posture of arrogance or a grimace on your face as you try to make it through the day, but as a natural result of feeling loved and confident?

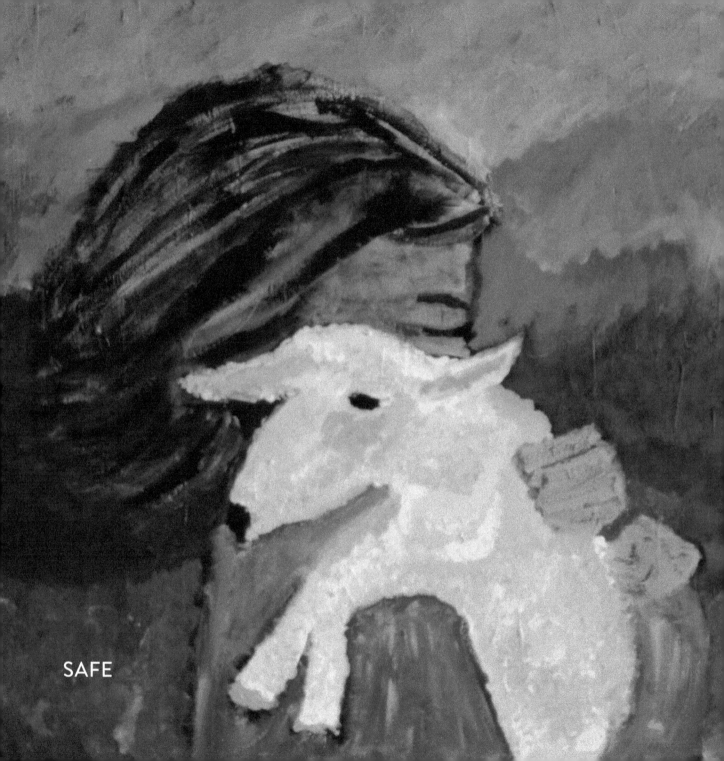

SAFE

16

Craving Safety

He tends his flock like a shepherd:
He gathers the lambs in his arms
and carries them close to his heart;
he gently leads those that have young.

(Isaiah 40:11)

I was sobbing on the phone with a stranger half the world away from me. I had gotten the phone number to Affair Recovery after discovering that many of the videos they had on YouTube gave words to my journey. Yet, things weren't getting better. My husband would make a commitment and I would feel hopeful as things seemed better for a while, just to find my world crashing down again as he resorted back to acting-out behaviors. As I described the ups and downs, this lady I didn't know told me, "Oh, I'm so very sorry. Ambivalence in spouses is so hard because they don't know what they want." She was so kind as she listened to me and told me where to find resources and help.

Rick Reynolds, the founder of Affair Recovery has this to say about ambivalence: "Ambivalence can also rock the world of the betrayed spouse. When their mate says they agree to give the marriage a chance, it instills hope. When they later say they have absolutely zero desire to work on saving the marriage, it's devastating. It's like experiencing whiplash while standing completely still."

We often see babies who have been crying calm down when they are picked up by a loved one. They recognize the smell and the embrace. They know they are safe. I longed for that feeling of safety.

The crazier my world seemed to get, the more I craved safety. I wanted to find that safe place. Yet, the world I knew seemed more and more full of uncertainty. I needed to feel secure. I became hypervigilant because I never knew what would be coming next. Being blindsided repeatedly led me to being fearful all the time. I needed to know I would be okay.

I needed to feel safe.

I sought safety in many ways.

Setting boundaries.
Seeking counseling.
Watching videos.
Listening to podcasts.
Reading books.
Praying more.
Reading my Bible.

I wanted our marriage back on firm ground so I could feel safe again.

Eventually, I had to let go of the expectation that my safety would come from my marriage.

I had to realize that my safety was in Jesus.

After painting this picture, I hung it up in my room where I could see it from my bed.

Daily I am reminded that I am a little lamb in the arms of Jesus.
Daily I remind myself that I can feel safe as I fall asleep at night.
Daily, I remind myself that I am safe for whatever comes ahead of me.

Questions *to* Consider:

1 When do you feel emotionally safe?

2 When does your safety feel threatened?

3 Are there steps you need to take to bring some stability to your life? Are there boundaries you need to set to experience safety?

4 Are you able to find emotional safety in the arms of Jesus? If not, do you know what is blocking this feeling of safety?

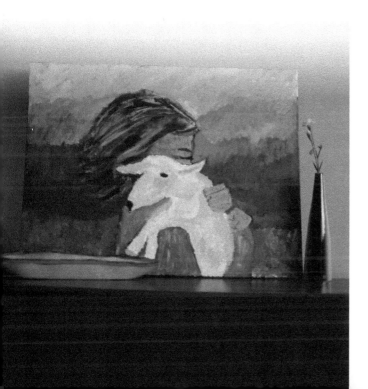

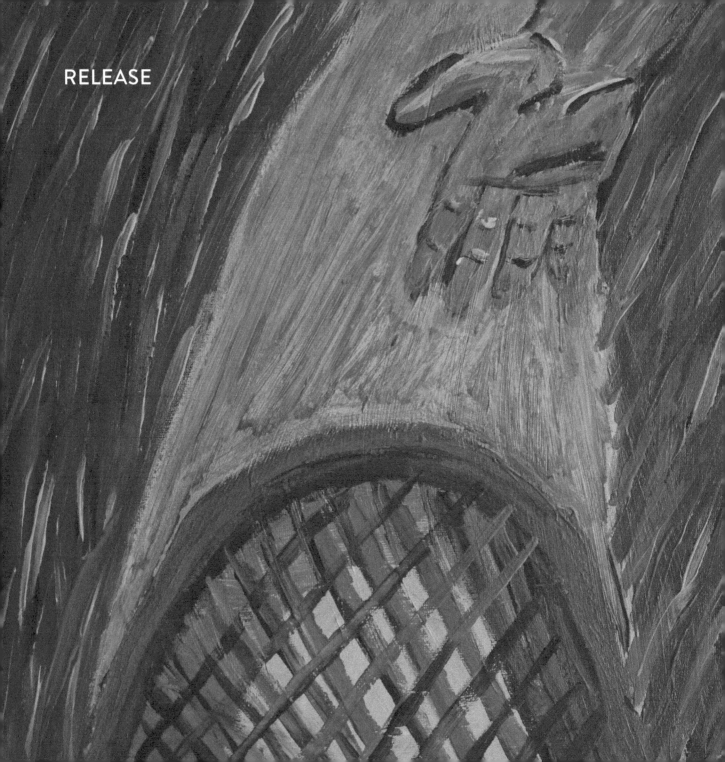

RELEASE

17

The Way it Should have been

But when she could hide him no longer, she got
a papyrus basket for him and coated it with tar
and pitch. Then she placed the child in it and put
it among the reeds along the bank of the Nile.

(Exodus 2:3)

Jochebed was placed in a horrible position. A healthy, wonderful baby boy was born to her, but the Egyptians were killing the Hebrew babies. So, she took her most treasured possession and put him in a basket made of reeds and tar. She bent down and released the basket into the Nile River.

We know the rest of the story. Pharaoh's daughter found the baby and raised him. Moses was safe.

But, at the time that Jochebed released her baby, she couldn't have known if it would end well or not. Pharaoh's daughter could have had the baby killed.

I clutched on to what I wanted for my life. I wanted to find the right information, the right program, or the right person to help. I worked very hard for years in a quest to find answers, resources and help. Something in me thought if I worked hard enough on it, I could find the answer to help and motivate my husband. I desperately wanted things to be the "way it should have been." It was the picture I had of a healthy Christian marriage.

One resource that was helpful for me was going through Marsha Means' Journey to Healing and Joy: A Workbook for Partners of Sexual Addicts. It was three years after D-Day before I was ready to go through this book.

In the first months after D-Day, I would have had a hard time going through this book because of the term "sexual addict." It's a label that seems hard to put on a loved one. I found many other terms during my research and counseling sessions that could have been used—approval addict, intimacy disorder or anorexia, or someone struggling with sexual compulsions and/or brokenness.

Eventually, I realized it didn't really matter what term was used.

The exact label of what to call someone who distances themselves from their own spouse and numbs themself with either actual or fantasy relationships with others may not matter, but it does help to put some language to some of these patterns. Regardless of the label, the actions leave a spouse reeling in the wake of betrayal.

I know our human tendency is to compare our spouse's actions to those of others. Sometimes we can think "at least he isn't nearly as bad as..." Other times, we realize that what we thought might have been a normal battle that every man faces, was actually something much more severe and should have caused red flags.

In my former husband's case, I wasn't sure what was caused by mental health and what was caused by sin. I simply knew that I was aching in pain. But, the truth was that his actions were killing our marriage and my image of an intimate, godly marriage. His behaviors outside of the marriage were eroding away what I believed about myself and the covenant of marriage.

I could see that in his mind there was some kind of moral justification or suspension for his actions, but they did not line up with his belief system. There was no way to completely understand his actions or the incredible grief and pain they brought to me.

In Marsha Means' Introduction to her workbook, she says, "Participation in such a group isn't dependent on how your husband has acted out sexually; what matters most is the deep searing pain you feel. As partners of these men, our lives have been turned upside down, and to heal, we have a journey of our own to take."

One of the first questions my mentor asked me as we began going through the workbook was what I wanted to gain by going through this time together. Immediately, I said, "I want to get off of this roller coaster."

My counselors had often told me that living in such an unpredictable environment was not sustainable. The familiar adage of "insanity is doing the same thing over and over again" was often repeated to me.

I was determined to find a way off the roller coaster that included my husband's clear thinking and his road to recovery. I wanted off the roller coaster, but I was only open to that happening by finding out the right person, counselor, program, Bible study, or accountability for my husband that would help him see his need for change.

Going through the workbook with a mentor helped me begin to see my powerlessness in getting my husband to do his recovery work. It helped me recognize that I couldn't make my husband make the choices that would make me feel safe.

I wasn't in control of his choice to cherish me and to fight for our marriage.

One person can't hold a two-person commitment together.

God was telling me it was time to let go.

I released my basket of dreams into the water.

Questions *to* Consider:

1 Is there anything in your life that God is asking you to release?

2 What pushback do you have to that idea? What are the costs that might come from releasing them? What are some benefits that might come from releasing?

3 Would release help you to get off of the roller coaster of ups and downs you may be on?

KEEP LOOKING UP

18
Looking Up

We do not know what to do, but our eyes are on you.

(2 Chronicles 20:12)

He says, "Be still, and know that I am God;
I will be exalted among the nations, I will be
exalted in the earth."

(Psalm 46:10)

I wonder how many puzzles I have put together in the last couple of years. Piece after piece. Flowers. Shelves of books. Doors.Waterfalls. City skylines. I needed for something to fit together. I have needed for pieces to make sense.

I like to know how things fit together.
What will come next..
I'm a planner.
A scheduler.
I love calendars and to-do lists.
I like formulas.
Equations with the same answer time after time.
And puzzles that end up looking like the picture on the box.

In my life, I look back and see how I thought I had done everything right. I thought I put the pieces together correctly.

I made wise choices in my dating life, remained a virgin, and married a Christian man who demonstrated similar values. We had Christian backgrounds where our parents and grandparents had marriages that lasted "til death parted them". We served in ministry together before we got married and continued to work in a church as soon as we got married. We both not only got along with our peers, but we loved children and senior citizens too. Our differences complemented each other well. We had similar backgrounds as we both grew up as missionary kids. We both brought

global perspectives into the marriage. None of our mentors or discipleship leaders or family members pointed out any red flags in our relationship.

My former husband was known for being humble, servant-hearted and kind. There were no "red flags."

According to the "formula" I had learned, ours was supposed to be a marriage that lasted.

I never put mental illness into the equation.

I had no understanding of hidden shame, obsessions, unwanted sexual behavior, or addictive habits.

I didn't know that, during the years of grappling with my husband's acting-out behaviors, I would live in a suspended place. A place of not knowing what to do or where to turn. So much of the time, I simply had no clue of how to respond.

None of the pieces fit together. Nothing made sense.

When all formulas failed me, the verse in 2 Chronicles 20:12 became a lifeline. Although there were counselors and podcasts and books, none of them could tell me what was exactly right for my journey. There was nothing that told me how long to keep fighting for my marriage. There was nothing that could tell me when it was time to let go.

Even though I did receive support, prayer and input from many sources, knowing what steps to take next came down to being between me and God.

It meant keeping my eyes on the Maker of heaven and earth.

Keeping in step with the Spirit.

Trusting God to show me the next right thing.

I wish I could tell others exactly what to do. That somehow through all of this, a neat little three-point list would have come to the surface that I could pass along to others. But, I'm learning that is not how life works. Yes, seek input and get advice from people who know you and love you and from experts in the field. Most importantly, keep looking up. Keep your eyes on the Creator. Trust Him to lead you one day at a time.

I found He was faithful to keep showing me what to do, one step at a time.

Questions *to* Consider:

1 Where do you usually turn when you don't know what to do?

2 Do you have people who are safe for you to talk to?

3 Have you found resources that have helped you on this journey?

4 Has listening to God made a difference for you? Are you able to see any gifts He has given you during this time?

5 How can you look up to Him today and listen to what He has to say?

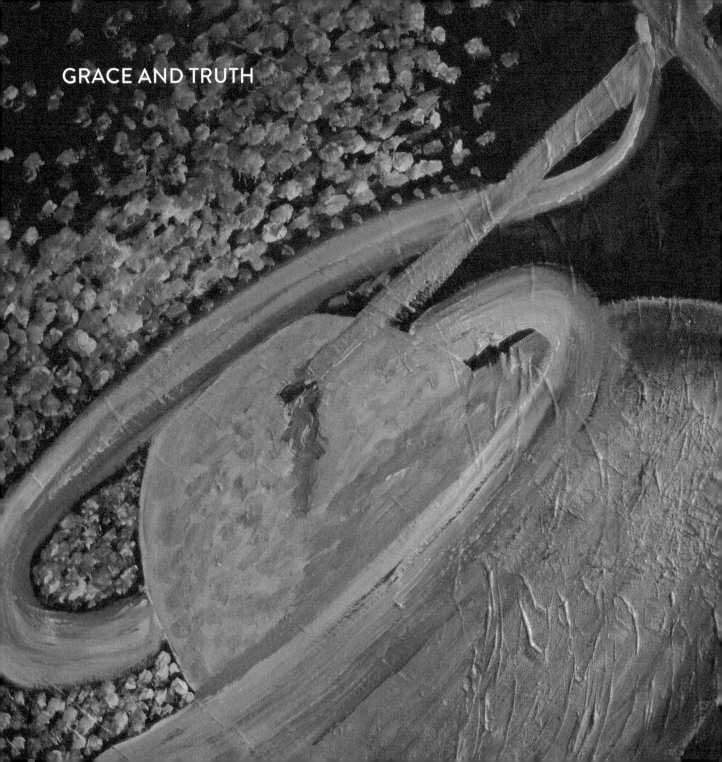

GRACE AND TRUTH

19

They Go Together

The Word became flesh and made his dwelling
among us. We have seen his glory, the glory of the
one and only Son, who came from the Father,
full of grace and truth.

(John 1:14)

Peanut butter and jelly.
Cookies and milk.
Macaroni and cheese.
Mangoes and sticky rice.

Some things just go together.

Grace and truth are like that, too.

If we only have grace, we will tend to overlook sin in ourselves and others. We will try to "get over it quickly" and move on with our lives. We will be compassionate, but nothing may change. We will forgive quickly and easily. We will want to put the hard stuff behind us and move on.

If we only have truth, we will call out sin quickly and easily. We may not have empathy. We will be quick to criticize. We will hold things against others. We will be so focused on behavior, that we will miss what was happening at a deeper level. We will be concerned about justice and punishment, rather than love and compassion.

If we have both, like Jesus did, they will work together beautifully.

Grace will surround us and give us the strength and ability to face the truth.

Truth will not always be pleasant but as it cuts into us, it will help us to heal.

When the pain of truth feels too hard to bear, grace will remind us there is love surrounding it and cushioning it.

I didn't realize how fond I was of denial. For most of my life, when things were hard I wanted to ignore the truth and pretend all was well. I so badly wanted everything to be okay. I wanted to move beyond anything unpleasant because I wanted to forgive and forget.

Unfortunately, that doesn't help get to the root of the problems.

I feel like God has helped me so much in the last few years to be able to see ugliness in myself and in others. I don't have to turn away from hard things or pretend like they don't exist. I'm able to face them and to know that God's grace covers them. I have to be able to see the bad in order to appreciate the grace.

It took both grace and truth to be able to look at my husband's actions accurately. Sometimes I wanted to deny the truth of the tremendous pain I was in and just go back to "being normal" for the sake of our family. That wasn't true grace because it ignored the truth. Sometimes I only wanted to look at the truth of his actions and think that he was a terrible person. That wasn't seeing Him with God's eyes of grace—the same grace that had forgiven me again and again.

As God opened my eyes to both grace and truth, I was able to see my husband more clearly as a sinner.

I was also able to love him even more deeply because I understood grace better.

Questions *to* Consider:

1 Do you tend to lean towards grace or truth in your relationships with others?

2 If your natural leaning is towards grace, what can you do to get a more objective view of your situation?

3 If your natural leaning is towards truth, what can you do to show more grace in your situation?

4 Since Jesus is full of both, spend some time with Him as you think about these two words. Be willing for the truth of the reality of the situation to pierce your heart. Take time to let grace surround your hurting heart, cushioning you and comforting you in the midst of your pain.

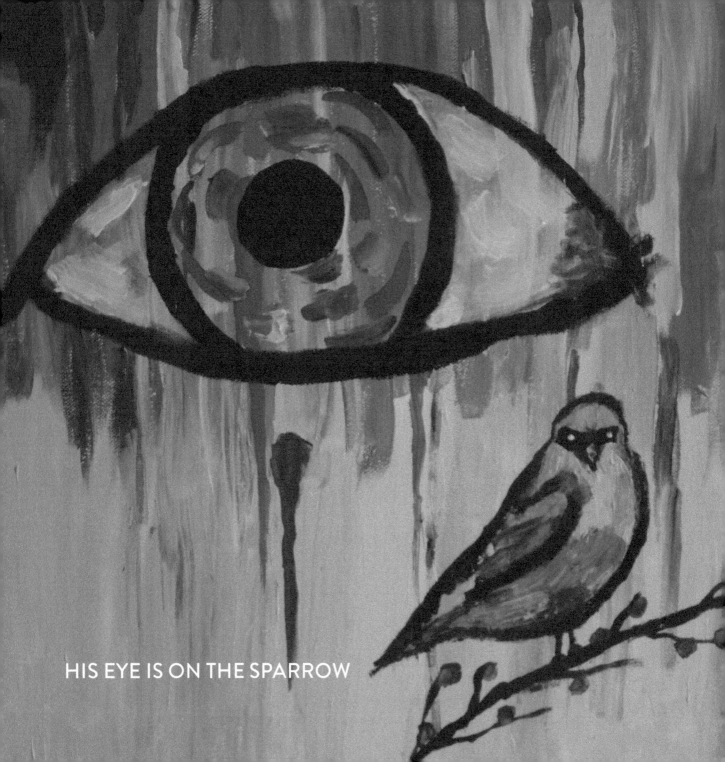

HIS EYE IS ON THE SPARROW

20

Alone
(But Not)

Are not two sparrows sold for a penny? Yet not
one of them will fall to the ground outside your
Father's care. And even the very hairs of your head
are all numbered. So don't be afraid; you are
worth more than many sparrows.

(Matthew 10:29-31)

Are not two sparrows sold for a penny? Yet not one of them will fall to the ground outside your Father's care. And even the very hairs of your head are all numbered. So don't be afraid; you are worth more than many sparrows. (Matthew 10:29-31)

After D-Day occurred, I had read statistics that if both partners were working hard on recovery, that the marriage could be restored to a new and better marriage within eighteen to twenty-four months. Sometimes it seemed like things were going well and I had so much hope that we were on that trajectory.

Then I would realize that, in some way or another, my husband wasn't committed completely to me. My desire to be the "one and only" woman in our marriage would suffer another crushing blow.

One night like that was New Year's Eve, 2018. It was the night before the dawn of another wedding anniversary that would bring sorrow instead of joy.

I wrote this poem about that experience.

Alone, But Not

I was alone that night as the new year came in.
One chair on the balcony.
One glass of sparkling juice.
One candle on a little table.
One lonely heart watching fireworks, fearful of another year.

And then, just one word.
Near.
I felt it whispered into my soul.
The Creator of the vast night sky and the Maker of my heart spoke to me.
I didn't have enough energy or initiative to ask for a word.
But,
He spoke it anyway.
And somehow my aching heart heard.
He was near.
He would be near.
The year would come.
More pain would come.
More tears would come.
But through it all, He would be here.
Beside me.
With me.
In me.
Near.

No matter how alone you may feel, I hope you know that God sees you and He is near.

Questions *to* Consider:

1. How has loneliness been part of your journey?

2. Why do you think it feels so lonely?

3. Who cares about you and wants to be a safe place for you to turn to? A good friend ? A counselor? God?

4. Think about the ways you can turn to those who are safe for you to be near to during this journey.

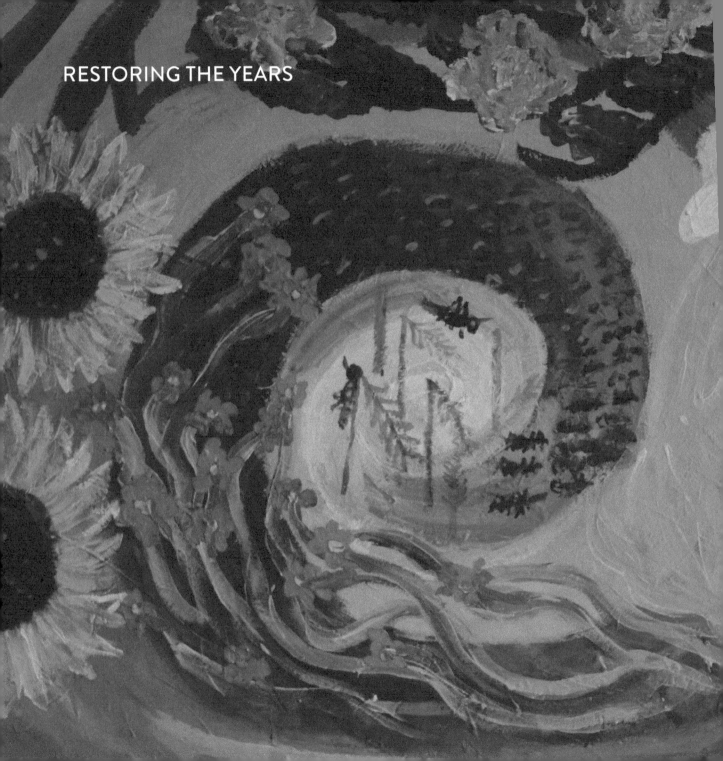

RESTORING THE YEARS

21

The Years the Locusts Have Eaten

I will repay you for the years the locusts have eaten—
the great locust and the young locust,
the other locusts and the locust swarm—
my great army that I sent among you.
You will have plenty to eat, until you are full,
and you will praise the name of the Lord your God,
who has worked wonders for you;
never again will my people be shamed.
Then you will know that I am in Israel,
that I am the Lord your God,
and that there is no other.

(Joel 2:25-27)

It felt like the locusts had devoured our family.

Our family that had been respected.
Our family once had the home where all the other teens hung out.
My own teens often told me that their friends said that they wished they had parents like us.

I remember when our first daughter went away to college and let us know how grateful she was for our family as she encountered many others who came from broken and dysfunctional homes. When my son went to college, I remember him sharing with me how other guys asked him how it was that he wasn't addicted to porn and he credited our home environment and our involvement in his life.

But, now, it seemed like everything good had been stripped away.

During this time, one of my daughters shared with me how a friend sent her these verses from Joel. On the same day when she turned to her Bible app, it had the same verses!

Then, that very week she found out that the town her Dad was working in was named Locust.

It seemed God was trying to tell us something.

As I thought more about these verses, I could picture growth and greenness spiraling backwards and replacing the years that the locusts had eaten.

Growth and beauty replacing the barrenness I felt.

That restoration is more than just "from this point on" God is bringing beauty.
It is a backwards restoration.
Flourishing in reverse.
It's otherworldly.
It is shame being lifted away from not just today, but from yesterday, too.
It's the very things that caused the pain now bringing forth something new.
It's the God of life.
The God of resurrection.

I long for the miracle of redemption. I long to see God bring beauty from this broken story.

Questions _to_ Consider:

1. What areas in your life and heart feel like they have been "eaten by locusts?"

2. Are you able to picture green flourishing in your life again? Why or why not?

3. Spend a few minutes in silence. Think about your future. Ask God for what He has in store for your life in the future. Does a picture come to your mind of healing and growth?

4. Do you find any encouragement in thinking your pain does not have to be wasted?

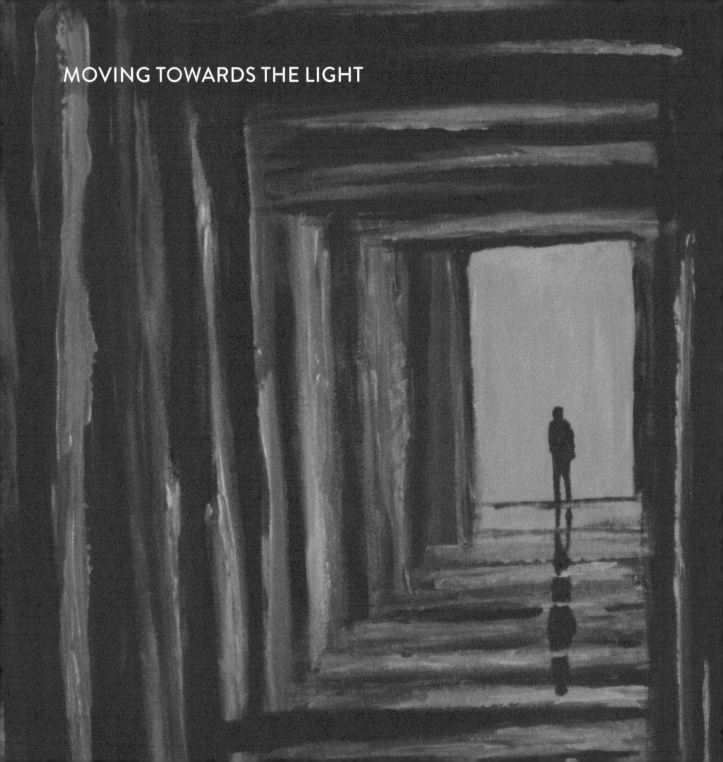

MOVING TOWARDS THE LIGHT

22

The Light is Already Shining

...because the darkness is passing and
the true light is already shining.

(1 John 2:8b)

When Jesus spoke again to the people, he said,
"I am the light of the world. Whoever follows
me will never walk in darkness, but will have
the light of life."

(1 John 2:8b)

When Jesus spoke again to the people, he said, "I am the light of the world. Whoever follows me will never walk in darkness, but will have the light of life." (John 8:12)

During one of my dark days, I came across a painting by Christy Marsh called "Light at the End of the Tunnel." It spoke to me. I was inspired to paint the image of someone walking through a dark tunnel to the light. Many days, it was easy to forget that the light was shining. All I could see was the darkness.

The grief of being alone and rejected ripped my heart into pieces. I had watched my mother travel through grief after becoming a widow. I saw her loneliness and how much she missed my Dad. I saw how her life was totally changed and how hard it was for her to lose her husband, the man she had loved for so long. I saw how difficult it was for her to figure out all the business-type of decisions that had to be made now that she was a widow. I realized how painful it was for her to do things alone.

I could relate on so many levels. I missed "the other half of me" and my best friend, too. I missed having someone to talk to and tell all about my day and to laugh at a million inside jokes. I missed the father of my children being around to rejoice in their victories and to pray through their struggles. I missed the million and one qualities he had that

drew people to him, like his kindness, his servant heart, and his sense of humor. I also had to learn to live as a single person. I also had to arrive at church alone. There were a multitude of financial and business decisions for me, too.

I know you can't compare grief and I am not trying to do that. I would like to share some of the differences of our grief, however, in hopes that the multiple layers of betrayal trauma and divorce are illustrated.

My mother had the comfort of a few things I didn't have. Her memories of their fifty-five years were not tainted. She can remember them with joy. She was left with knowing how much my Dad loved her and how he delighted in her. His eyes sought her out wherever she was, even when he could not move any other parts of his body. She had the comfort of people remembering his godliness and the impact he had made on their lives. During anniversaries, birthdays and holidays, friends would write in with memories, pictures and encouragement. Her grief was recognized and responded to with love and support.

I was left with the realization that my husband didn't love me enough. His own narrative of our life together was so different from what I thought our marriage had been that I didn't know if he had ever loved me in the way I had believed. Pictures of our life together brought pain. Memories of our three years of dating and thirty years of marriage were emotionally charged. I didn't know how to tell others about the death of our marriage.

I listened to Jason Gray's song "Death Without a Funeral" on repeat. HIs song describes the way divorce does not get the closure and grief that physical death brings.

His lyrics spoke to my pain in the dark.

But light does penetrate darkness.

Jesus had already brought light into our dark world and the light was already shining. I had to be willing to look for it. To keep putting one foot ahead of the other on a quest to find it. To immerse myself in worship music and scripture and friends who reminded me of the truth.

I had to look for a flicker of light in the smile of a friend. Or a soft glow as I looked at a sunset.

The light was already shining. I just needed to keep moving towards it.

Questions *to* Consider:

1. Think about the things that bring light into your life. Make a list—perhaps these ideas might help your thoughts to get going!

- a great conversation with a friend
- hot chocolate or an ice cream cone
- spending time in creation—at a waterfalls, beach, or in your own yard
- watching a sunrise or sunset
- spending time in God's Word
- the smile of your baby or grandbaby
- the smell of your favorite flower or meal
- your favorite worship song

2. Spend some time thanking your Creator for the gifts in your life that help you remember His light.

3. What are some things you can do to remember and recognize God's light in your life this week?

4. If you begin to get swallowed up in darkness, remind yourself that Jesus is the Light. Take some time to focus on Him and the gifts He has given you.

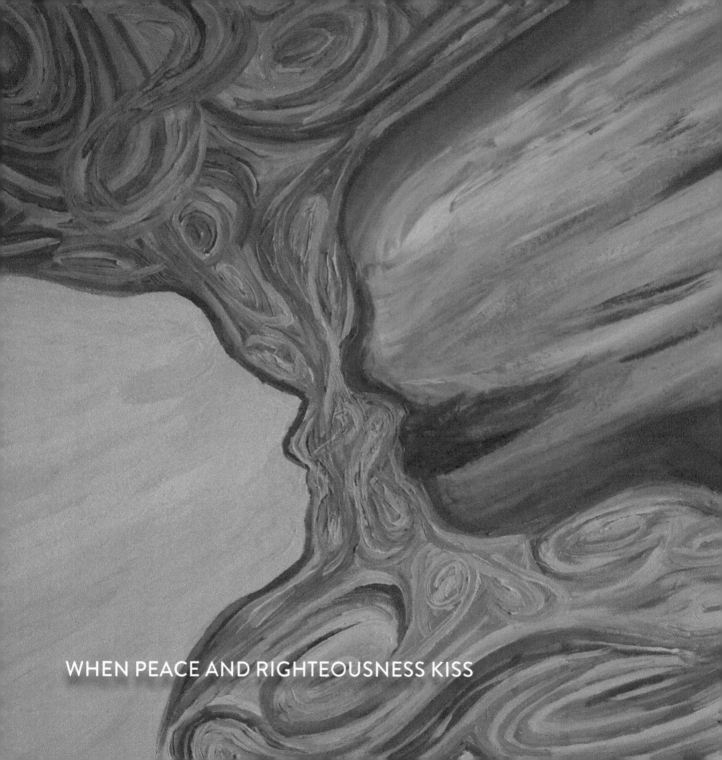

WHEN PEACE AND RIGHTEOUSNESS KISS

23

Kisses

Love and faithfulness meet together;
righteousness and peace kiss.

(Psalm 85:10)

I was thirsty for stories of hope, healing, and restoration. I watched videos, read books and listened to podcasts. I heard stories of husbands who had hurt their wives deeply, but they truly repented and did the hard work of recovery. Time and time again, I saw couples who said, "Now our relationship is better than it has ever been. We have learned to go to deeper levels in our communication. We've seen each other's sins and weaknesses, and, yet, we love and treasure each other more."

The stories gave me hope. I soaked up every helpful tip about addiction and healing and recovery. I kept thinking we were headed in that direction, too. Commitments would be made that sounded good. I felt like I was loving my husband better as we had hard conversation after hard conversation.

I understood that sexual addiction was not some strange, deranged type of thinking. Instead, it simply referred to those who used fantasy and other sexual escapes to try to avoid pain in life. I learned that we all turn to coping habits to self-soothe.

Sometimes, those self-soothing behaviors are harmful.

Jonathan Daugherty, in his book Secrets says "Sexual addiction really is about escape, running away from all that is not comfortable or convenient. There is certainly more to it in terms of its complexity and how it manifests itself in different people, but ultimately it drives a person to escape pain. What the sex addict doesn't understand, however, is that continuing to medicate the pain with secret sexual behaviors only increases the agony. In my attempt to escape pain, I only invited more in."

I understood escape and could have compassion on my husband. I also turn to escapes such as social media, reading, and food. Even though my husband's actions hurt and angered me, I could understand what was behind the actions. I could work on my love being more mature and complete—not based on what I wanted, but learning to love him even knowing where he turned to in order to hide his own pain.

Yet, as the months and years went by, it didn't look like our marriage was going to end in restoration. Instead, I was alone in my apartment. I was grappling with deep loss and with the awareness that it was time to let go.

One night, I was listening to the book of Psalms as I tried to fall asleep. This verse about righteousness and peace kissing woke me up! I had never noticed it before.

My world had changed from being in an intimate relationship to suddenly being in a world without any kisses.

I needed this picture of a God whose world is full of kisses.

Righteousness and peace.
Love and faithfulness.
Truth and grace.
Faithfulness and truth.
Sorrow and delight.
Heaven and earth.

This painting was pure joy to swirl on canvas. I loved thinking about the God who even kisses with colors, combining yellow and blue to make green!

Questions *to* Consider:

1 How does your heart respond to the idea that righteousness and peace kiss? How could this union look in your situation?

2 Are there any other two concepts that are important for you to pair together?

3 Do you relate to Jonathan Daugherty's quote about sexual addiction being an escape from all that is not comfortable and convenient? Have you seen this to be true in you or your loved one's story?

4 What are areas of healthy escape for you? What areas of escape only bring about more problems?

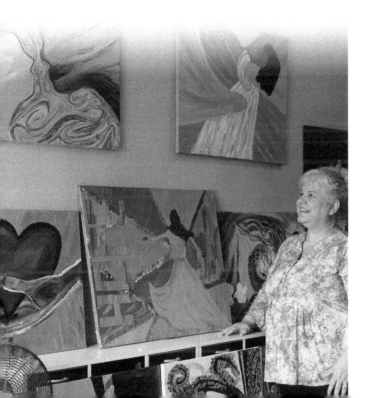

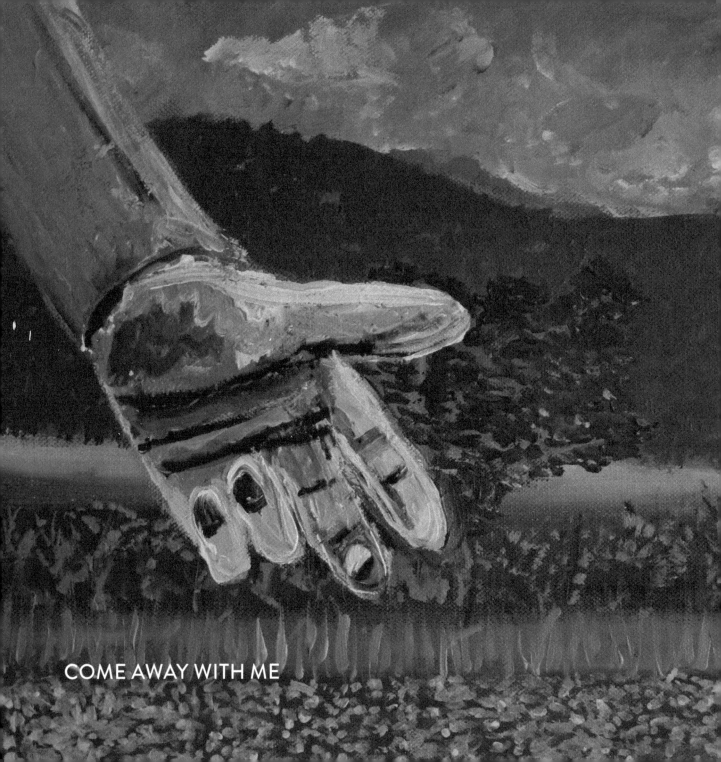

COME AWAY WITH ME

24

Pace, Space
and Grace

Then, because so many people were coming and
going that they did not even have a chance to eat,
he said to them, "Come with me by yourselves to
a quiet place and get some rest."

(Mark 6:31)

This is what the Sovereign Lord, the Holy One of
Israel, says: "In repentance and rest is your salvation,
in quietness and trust is your strength.

(Isaiah 30:15)

If you are injured in a car crash or diagnosed with cancer, it is obvious you need to slow down in order to concentrate on healing. You may be in the hospital or severely limited in what you have the capacity to do. You may be limited physically in a way that changes your former schedule. Most likely, you have to make adjustments to your life as you give time for healing.

With D-Day, it was obvious that all was not well in our marriage. Our marriage was extremely important to me and I knew we needed to scale back and reschedule our lives. As therapy and counseling took much of our time and resources, we had to adjust to a new pace. As I realized my husband felt like I didn't listen to him, I resolved to do better. I wanted a schedule where we had time to connect daily. It was necessary to cut back on a lot in our lives in order to concentrate on our relationship.

I read books and listened to podcasts that suggested that with work, marriages could heal. Then, after a couple of years of hard work, when my husband and counselor said I was doing too much work and not enough play or laughter, I tried to make space in our schedule for that, too. We upped our dating game and took more trips together.

Leaving space in our lives for downtime and fun time was important. I also needed more space for reflection as I tried to examine my heart and tried to become more self-aware. I needed time to learn about addiction and restoration.

I learned, though, that I couldn't heal by just "trying harder." It also became obvious that trying harder didn't mean that the sexual brokenness issues disappeared. It often made it more painful when slip-ups and relapses happened, because I knew I was making positive changes in myself, but his behaviors were not changing.

I learned that marriage can only be as healthy as the least healthy person.

I couldn't hold the marriage together by myself, but I could keep working on my inner world.

In order to heal, I needed to give up control.
To slow down more.
To let go more.
To learn to take care of myself. Not in a selfish way, but in a way that identified what my heart and body needed. Then, I needed to spend time with God to allow Him to show me how those needs could be met.

I also had to let go of the goal of reconciliation and instead have the goal of being at rest with God.

I had to remind myself to receive God's grace.
I had to give myself grace.

After my husband left, one of my mentors challenged me to take a trip on my own. It seemed intimidating and overwhelming. My life had revolved around marriage and family for so long. I wasn't sure I could enjoy a trip by myself.

As I prayed about it, I felt God was inviting me to come away with Him. Not alone, but with Him by my side. I made arrangements to spend a few days in Khao Yai. I painted this while looking out my window.

It ended up being a sweet step in my healing journey.

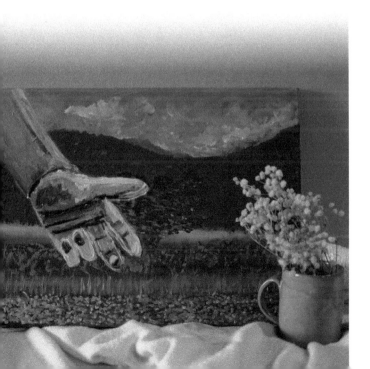

Questions *to* Consider:

1 Have you been able to give yourself permission for quietness and rest?

2 What are some steps you could take to slow down your pace of life?

3 Are you able to identify some areas where your body and heart could use some care? What are some steps you could take for self-care?

4 Are there areas you are expecting too much of yourself right now? What would it look like to offer yourself some grace?

5 Try to find some creative ways to "come away and rest" so that God's Spirit has time and space to refresh you.

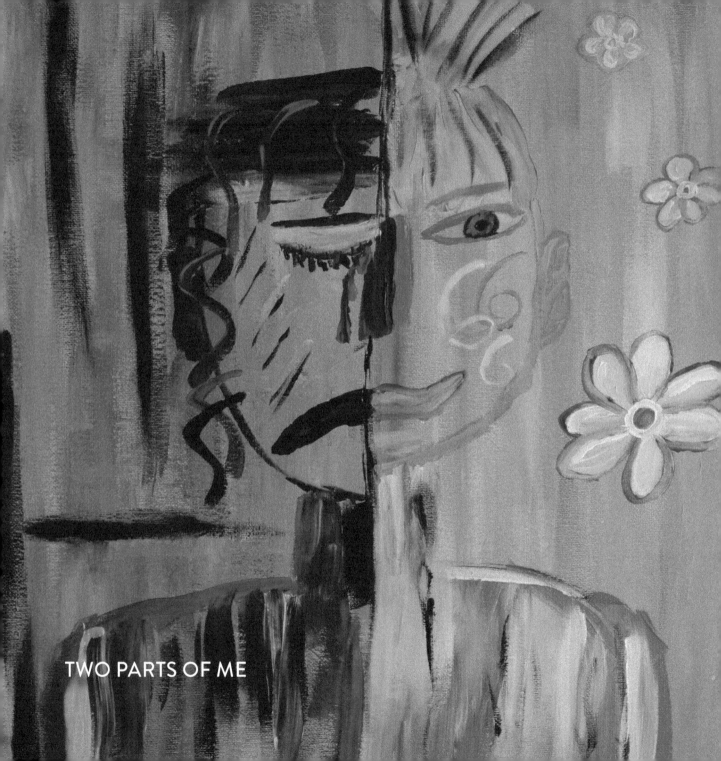

TWO PARTS OF ME

25

The Real Me

For whatever is hidden is meant to be
disclosed, and whatever is concealed is meant
to be brought out into the open.

(Mark 4:22)

I had never had any problem with being the real me. I'm one of those people whose face is an open book. I valued openness and authenticity. I didn't have things to hide so it was easy to be transparent.

Then I found myself in a story with things I didn't know how to put words to.

A story with hiddenness.
A story with shame.
A story of choices that left me feeling humiliated.

I remember early on in the journey, my counselor telling me I would need some "inner circle" people with whom I would be safe sharing my story. She said there would be others whom I could give a general idea of how things were going, and there would be those in the outer circle who just didn't need to know.

It was exhausting and disconcerting to go out in public. How did I even answer a simple question like "how are you?"

It seemed like there were minefields around every bend.

I wanted to honor my husband. I wanted to protect him while we tried to find something that would help him heal. This meant I felt like I couldn't share his weaknesses. How I wished he left his socks on the floor or that he left the toilet lid up or something else that was less severe to share, rather than the reality of why our marriage was struggling.

I hated feeling hypocritical.

I had to take deep breaths before I could walk into any room.

Sometimes my therapist would help me come up with a phrase I could repeat when people asked me questions.

I learned the art of deflection and shifting the conversation onto the other person.

At work, I needed to be professional. I couldn't lie in a fetal position, weeping.

Having two parts of me was painful. It wasn't what I wanted.

I do believe it has given me more empathy and understanding for others who, for one reason or another, feel compelled to hide part of their story. It reminds me of the iceberg principle and that we often are only seeing just a part of other people and not the deeper parts hidden beneath the surface.

I'm still wrestling with this, even as I paint and write. How much do I disclose? What is helpful to others and what is unnecessary?

I pray that God will give me the courage to share my story in a way that is honest and real and, yet, sensitive towards others.

Questions *to* Consider:

1 Do you identify with feeling like two parts of you are in tension with each other?

2 What are ways you are being honest about yourself and your story, even if you feel like you cannot disclose everything?

3 Do you get anxious about answering questions that other people ask? What are some things you could do to help with this?

4 Your true emotions and responses are valuable. Who are you able to share the deepest parts of your heart with? Can you stop and share your real thoughts and feelings with God right now?

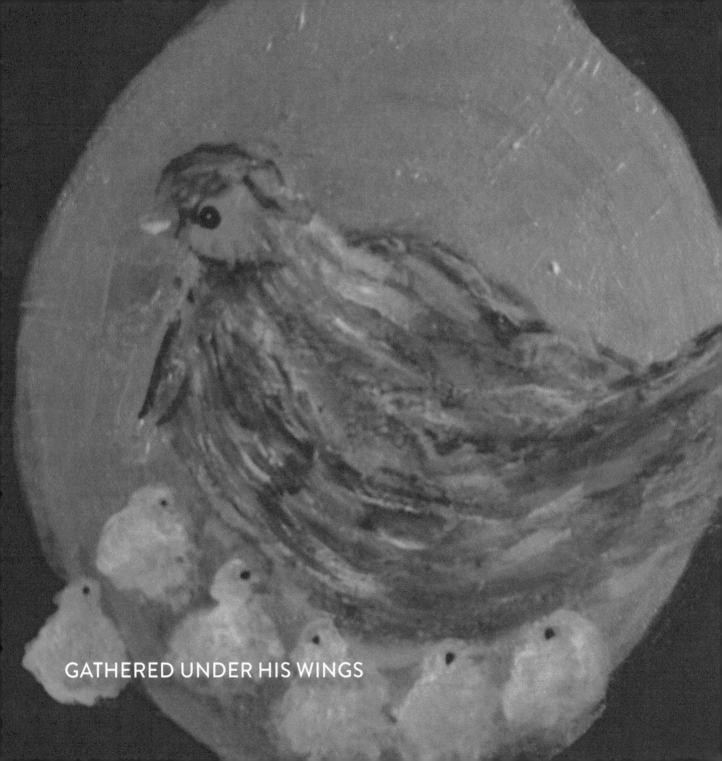

GATHERED UNDER HIS WINGS

26

Comforted

Jerusalem, Jerusalem, you who kill the prophets and
stone those sent to you, how often I have longed to
gather your children together, as a hen gathers her
chicks under her wings and you were not willing.

(Matthew 23:37)

He will cover you with his feathers,
and under his wings will you find refuge.

(Psalm 91:4)

One of my favorite movies is the Emma Thompson adaptation of Jane Austen's Sense and Sensibility. Whenever I could tell that my husband still didn't "get it" the following scene would replay in my head.

Elinor Dashwood: Whatever his past actions, whatever his present course... at least you may be certain that he loved you.
Marianne: But not enough. Not enough.

It was difficult to realize that my husband didn't love me enough to fight for our marriage and to work on his issues.

There were times I would just look at him, trying to find the man I knew. He would ask, "Why are you looking at me like that?" And, I would tearfully tell him I was trying to find him again. This man holding on so hard to what he wanted was so different from the man I had known whose heart had been so tender to the Lord and to me.

And, later, it was hard to come to grips with the fact that the time of fighting for the marriage was over for me and that it was time to let go. Everything in me rebelled against this because I was pretty sure it would end in losing the marriage and the relationship that had meant so much to me. Even though I was so hurt, I still wanted my husband to choose healing and restoration.

Although I had a good support group of family, friends and counselors, I still felt so alone.
I was the one losing the person with whom I had shared so many memories for over thirty years.
I was the one losing the dreams I had had for my future.
I was the one waking up alone in bed.

At an extremely low point, I asked God to show me that he saw me and cared about me. At this time, very few people knew that my husband had left me. Because of the pandemic and lockdown in our city, it wasn't very noticeable that we weren't together. I asked God very specifically that he would speak to someone who didn't know anything about our situation and ask them to pray for us. I wish I could say I prayed my request with great faith. Instead, it was more of a challenge to God, telling him I knew He had done things like that before in my past. It was crying out, letting Him know that I needed something. It was an entreaty that I needed validation and encouragement. It was a cry to know that I was seen and heard.

A couple of days later, my Mom called me. She shared that one of her retired missionary friends had called and said, "What is happening with Sheila and her husband?" When my Mom shared our situation with her, she said she knew it was something big and heavy because of the burden God put on her heart.

I'm so thankful for the tangible comfort God gave me that day.
I was not forgotten.
I was gathered under His feathers, and in His wings, I found refuge.

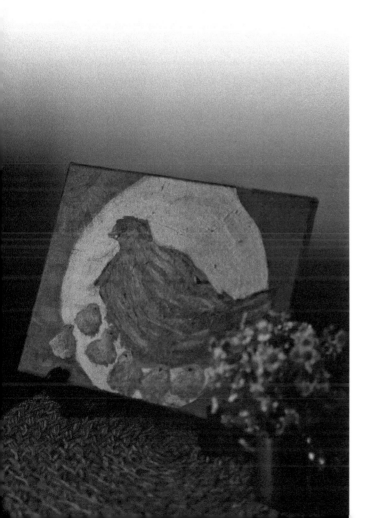

Questions *to* Consider:

1. Take a few minutes to watch some mother hen and little chicks videos on YouTube. Notice how the chicks stay so close to their mothers so that they can hide under their wings when danger comes. What are some ways you can walk closely with God?

2. Is your soul crying out to God about any specific areas...wanting to be seen? Comforted? Valued?

3. God is big enough for us to pour out our hearts before Him. Spend some time letting Him know your needs today.

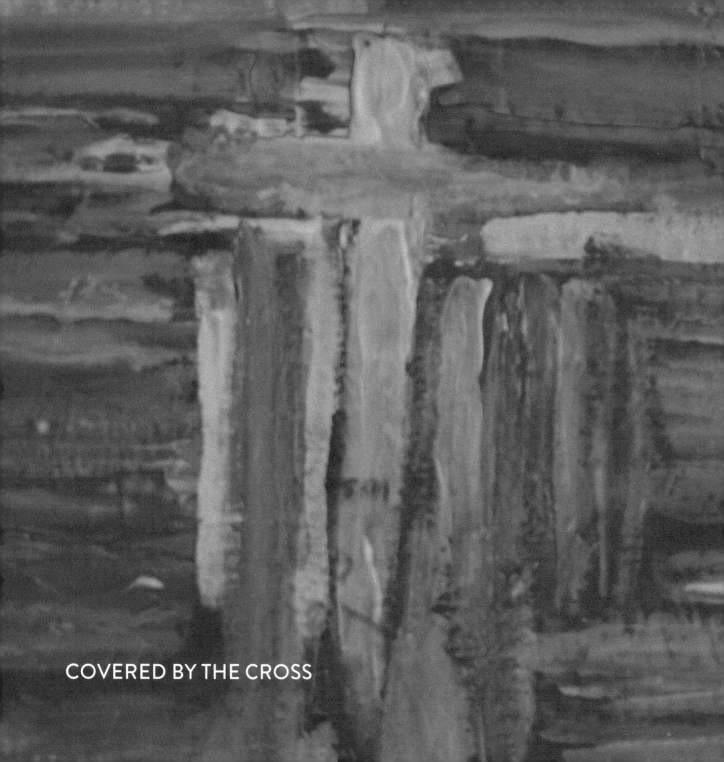

COVERED BY THE CROSS

27

Two Sinners in every Marriage

For all have sinned and fall
short of the glory of God.

(Romans 3:23)

I was certainly a sinner in my marriage.

I came with my own baggage.
I came with a desire to have our home be exactly what I dreamed it would be.
I wanted my husband to measure up to what I had dreamed of in a Christian husband.
I didn't have a good grasp of the fact that we would both be sinful and selfish every day, and that we would need the gospel to give us the grace we needed with each other.

As I've matured and grown in the grace and knowledge of God, His kindness has often led me to repentance. I discovered I had idols of comfort, stability, and reputation. Even idols of marriage and family. I saw that I clung to denial about the ugly things in life in myself and my loved ones because I didn't want to deal with disappointment.

As my marriage crumbled around me, I found that my husband had held back a lot of his thoughts about me. In order to keep the peace, he had withheld a lot of his feelings. He found me controlling, selfish, and a poor listener.

I've had to sift through those accusations. Of course, many of them are true. At my core, I am selfish and I do desire for life to go as I want it. I've had to take responsibility and ownership for being selfish and insensitive.

At the same time, because my husband didn't communicate many of his feelings to me, I have had to acknowledge that some things I couldn't work on because they required communication and negotiation and I simply didn't know they were causing injury. I had no idea that his resentments had built up for years. Therefore, I couldn't work on those areas until I was told about them.

After D-Day, I discovered even more of my sinful nature.
I discovered that I could feel rage.
I learned that when my emotions were flooding, I could say things in my anger I never believed I would say.
I discovered that I wanted to inflict pain on my husband so he would know what it felt like to be hurt so badly.
That sarcasm and unkindness were lurking beneath the surface of my heart.

It was important to me to keep going back to the cross. A prayer from the Episcopal Book of Common Prayer has been meaningful to me: "Most merciful God, we confess that we have sinned against you in thought, word, and deed, by what we have done and by what we have left undone. We have not loved you with our whole heart; we have not loved our neighbors as ourselves. We are truly sorry and humbly repent. For the sake of your Son Jesus Christ, have mercy on us and forgive us."

The beauty is that God does forgive us.

I've had to confess and repent repeatedly.

I've also had to choose to believe to live in the freedom of forgiveness.

I painted this depiction for an illustration to the teenagers I work with. I made a list of my many sins and wounds (judgment, pride, anger, bitterness, shame, anxiety, insecurity, etc.) I then painted the cross over all the words as an example of how Jesus has covered up my sins and forgiven me.

In owning my own sins, I also had to realize that my husband's unfaithful choices were not my fault.

They were about him and the decisions he made.

Just as he was not to blame for my sin, I was not to blame for his sin.

As I continually examine my heart, I find that in repentance, I can receive grace.

Questions *to* Consider:

1 What are some areas in your heart where you can see your issues, your sin, and your own emotional "baggage"?

2 As you acknowledge those, are you able to receive the healing and forgiveness that is offered through the cross?

3 If you are in a relationship with an unfaithful spouse, what are decisions and choices your spouse has made where the blame is not yours?

4 What are steps you can take in owning your own sin while not taking on the blame for the sins of others?

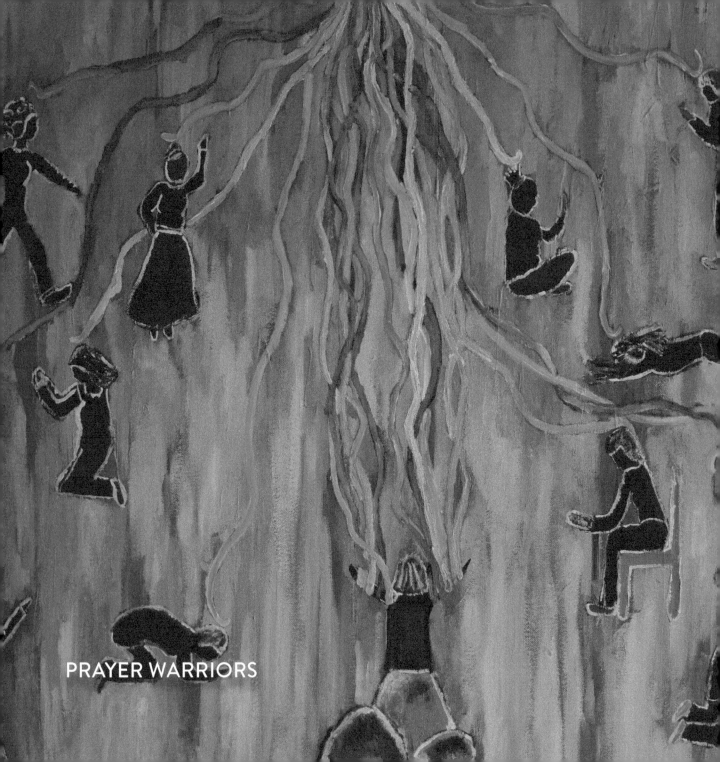

PRAYER WARRIORS

28

Held Up

So Joshua fought the Amalekites as Moses had ordered, and Moses, Aaron and Hur went to the top of the hill. As long as Moses held up his hands, the Israelites were winning, but whenever he lowered his hands, the Amalekites were winning. When Moses' hands grew tired, they took a stone and put it under him and he sat on it. Aaron and Hur held his hands up—one on one side, one on the other—so that his hands remained steady till sunset. So Joshua overcame the Amalekite army with the sword.

(Exodus 17:10-13)

Somehow, I continued breathing.
Getting up in the mornings.
Working.

I knew that I couldn't be doing it on my own.
On my own, I just wanted to stay in my bed forever.

In addition to my husband's betrayal and my son's suicide, I had also had a host of other losses in the same five-year time-frame. My father had died of a neurological disease, and it was so hard to watch as my once-strong surgeon Dad became unable to do the simplest of tasks as his body shut down on him. My cousin's beautiful nineteen-year-old daughter passed away after a heroic response to cancer over a span of six years. My son and his wife lost a baby through miscarriage. My father-in-law and mother-in-law both passed away. My nephew, in a completely unrelated incident to my own son's, took his own life due to mental health issues. This happened the day after my son's suicide, so our family had two heartbreaking funerals in one week.

Sometimes the losses seemed more than I could bear.

A couple of friends praying for me mentioned how the story of Aaron and Hur holding up Moses' arms had come to mind as they prayed for me.

An image came to my mind when they shared this.
I could see my friends praying...
Some who prayed while they took their evening walk.
Some who used prayer apps.
Some who prayed through the Bible.
Some who prayed daily with their husbands.
Some praying while they did their morning yoga.

Old women and young women.
Friends and family who loved me and who knew my world had been torn apart.

As I thought about their prayers, I could picture their prayers ascending to God's ear as ribbons. And, God lowering back the ribbons to hold up my arms.

I always thought I couldn't handle it if I encountered suicide or divorce in my life. Yet, within a couple of years, my son and my nephew took their lives. My husband had left me and divorce was looming in the future.

Yet, somehow, thanks to the prayers of friends and the grace of God, I was being held up.

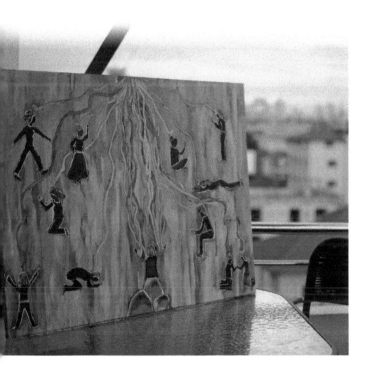

Questions *to* Consider:

1 Do you have people who are praying for you?

2 If so, spend some time today in gratitude for this blessing. Maybe you could let them know how much their prayers mean to you!

3 If not, do you have one or two trustworthy friends you could meet with this week to share part of your story and to invite them to pray for you?

4 Is God asking you to be a prayer warrior for someone else who is going through grief in their life?

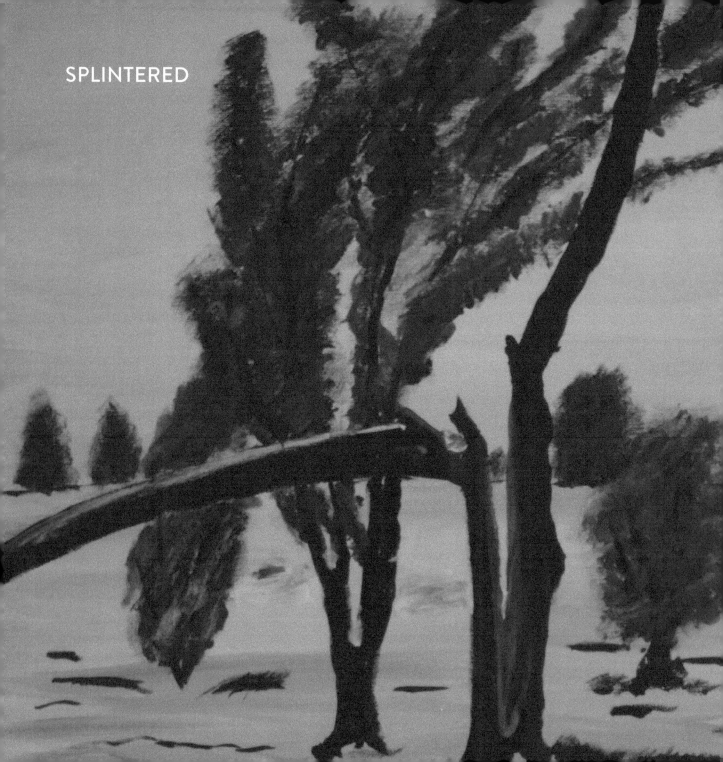
SPLINTERED

29

The Things God Hates

There are six things the Lord hates,
seven that are detestable to him:

naughty eyes,
a lying tongue,
hands that shed innocent blood,
a heart that devises wicked schemes,
feet that are quick to rush into evil,
a false witness who pours out lies
and a person who stirs up conflict in the community.

(Proverbs 6:16-19)

I gave faithless Israel her certificate of divorce and sent her
away because of all her adulteries.

(Jeremiah 3:8)

I've heard that God hates divorce for most of my life. As someone who was always the good little girl who wanted to do everything right, I knew I never wanted to participate in something that God hated. I grew up hearing the humorous phrase attributed to Ruth Bell Graham, Billy Graham's wife. When she was asked if she had ever considered divorce, she replied, "Divorce? No. Murder? Yes."

Divorce was unthinkable to me.

I was always told to never let divorce be part of my vocabulary and I kept that mindset for the first thirty years of my marriage. Even after D-Day and discovering the lies and betrayal, my heart's desire was for my husband to repent and walk in integrity and for our marriage to be restored. I wanted for us to do whatever work that needed to be done for reconciliation to happen.

Four and a half years beyond D-Day, when my husband walked out and said it was too hard to be married to me, I still didn't want to pursue divorce. I knew that boundaries had been broken and I needed to follow through on the consequences I had set for my safety. I started by pursuing legal separation. In talks with lawyers, I found that legal separation wasn't a viable option. It wasn't recognized in Thailand where I lived, or in my resident state. With urging from lawyers and godly mentors and counselors, I began pursuing divorce.

How could I walk towards something that God hated?

One reason was that I realized that God also hated patterns of deception.

Another was that I realized a marriage that reflected God's love for the church did not include a spouse who hid things and returned to acting-out behaviors repeatedly. I knew that I didn't want to enable a cycle of hidden sins.

I also knew that I was legalizing what had already taken place. My husband had repeatedly made choices that showed he did not want to be in a marriage with me, and he eventually walked out on me as I sobbed and begged him to stay.

There came a time when I knew God was telling me the best way to show love to my husband was by letting go and allowing him to make his own decisions. Not out of punishment or anger, but because in releasing, I was giving up control.

I was trusting God with my husband's life.

I still believe that God hates divorce.
I hate it, too.
I hate that our family is broken.
I hate that it feels like I have been torn in two.
I hate that we are not the picture of Christ and His bride the way that Christian marriage was intended.

I hate that the person I shared my life with and have a million memories and inside jokes with is no longer a part of my life.

I hate that the person whom I have loved for so long is not here to enjoy our children and grandchildren and empty nest years with me.

I hate that there is so much grief to work through daily.

I hate looking at thirty-three years of pictures and feeling such deep pain.

I hate that our children have parents who are not together and that they have to negotiate with both whenever they are planning weddings or vacations or holidays.

I believe that divorce is caused by sin.

I also believe that the sin can be hidden to those who are not close to the situation.

I think that it is easy to see the person who initiated the divorce as the one who sinned.

But sometimes, the divorce is a response to sin that has already been happening for a long time.

Often, it is a final separation away from a sinful and toxic pattern that is not pleasing to God.

Divorce should never be taken lightly. It is important that we try everything we can do to save our marriages. Godly counselors, mentors, friends, family, and our church leadership should be listened to during the process. It's important to cling to God's Word and to walk in obedience to Him. In doing that, there may come a time when God lets us know it is time to let go.

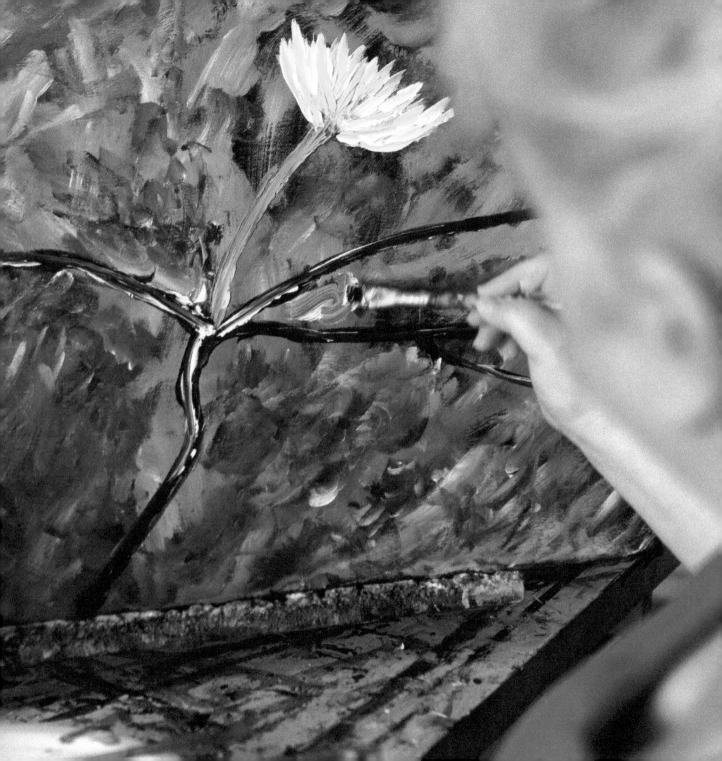

Questions *to* Consider:

1 What are your responses to the word "divorce"? Where do your responses come from?

2 If your spouse has done something that has broken the marriage covenant, do you believe God is asking you to pursue reconciliation? What steps have you taken and what other steps can you take towards restoration?

3 There are many nuances and "gray areas" for why someone might pursue divorce. While some lines that are crossed we might all agree on as reasons for a spouse to initiate divorce (child abuse, murder, physical affair) there are others that may not seem as clearly defined, such as repeated pornography viewing, hidden flirtatious texts to others, or property destroyed in anger. What are some examples you can think of where you would support a friend if they felt that they needed to initiate a divorce? In your own marriage, what would be a deal breaker for you?

4 Of course, even if someone has committed the very worst of offenses, there are occasions where they are truly repentant and willing to change and to pursue reconciliation and restitution. Would you be willing to pursue reconciliation if your spouse was truly repentant?

5 Ask God to show you His heart for you in your situation. Ask Him to give you the wisdom and discernment you need.

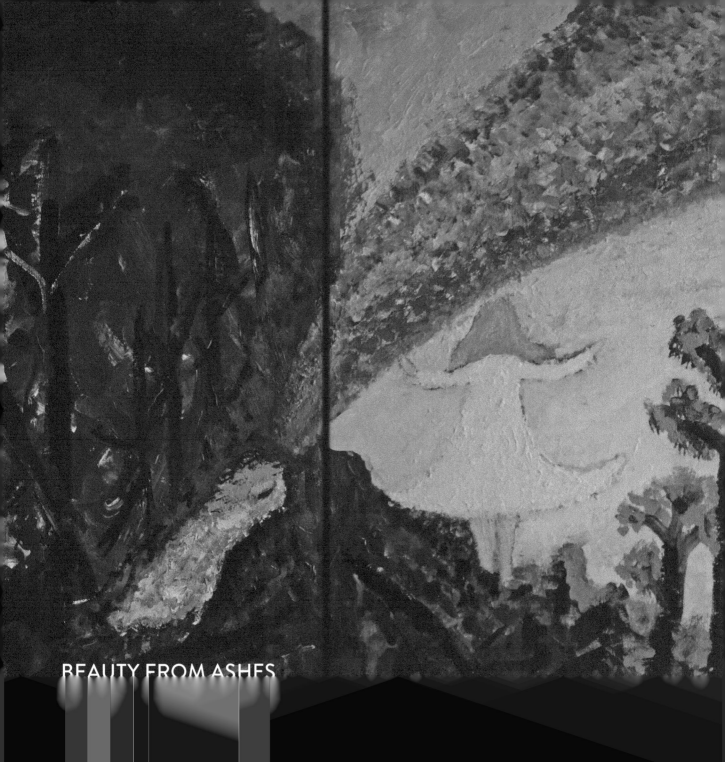

BEAUTY FROM ASHES

30

In The
Ashes

...to comfort all who mourn,
and provide for those who grieve in Zion—
to bestow on them a crown of beauty
instead of ashes,
the oil of joy
instead of mourning,
and a garment of praise
instead of a spirit of despair.

(Isaiah 61:3)

A few days after D-Day, I wrote this poem:

Grace in the Ashes

Today I sat in the heap of ashes
Even the good memories seemed gray.
If I tried to remember and hold on to them
They simply blew away.

Today, I tasted dusty ashes
The bitterness caused me to cry
With every bite, my lips choked out
The anguished question "why?"

Today, covered in soot and ashes,
I asked God to lift my head.
And to bestow a crown of beauty
To my soul that felt so dead.

Today, still colored gray in ash,
God kindly cupped my face.
He wept with me as He saw my pain,
Each teardrop bringing grace.

I felt like I was living in a gray world and that I might never feel alive or see beauty again.

I painted this two-canvas set over four years later after my husband left.

I still felt like I was in the ashes. The months since D-Day had been so hard.
I kept thinking that my husband would begin his healing process.

In fact, over and over again I thought there were indications he was on a healing path.
He met weekly in one-on-one meetings with other men.
He attended online support groups.
He had made it through one online course and was going through another.
He had gone to retreats, counseling, and even a residential treatment program.
He was taking his medication.

Yet, it seemed like he was still white-knuckling it and trying on his own strength. He still seemed to think he could try harder and become a person who kept his commitments. He wasn't trustworthy, yet he seemed to think that he was.

After listening to stories of so many men who had made significant changes, I could see he was not there, yet. Samson Society is an organization to help men come out of isolation and help each other. The founder of the Samson Society, Nate Larkin freely shares about his sex addiction and healing journey. Nate has said about his wife "She trusts me now because I don't trust myself."

I felt like the same cycles would continue until my husband could get to the point where he realized he needed help from others and he could share his deepest heart with others and let them help him on the journey.

I had been in the ashes a long time and I wanted to believe there would be a day when there is beauty again.

Questions *to* Consider:

1 Have you ever felt like you were in the heap of ashes and there was no beauty left in life?

2 Do you believe there will come a day when there is beauty again?

3 Take time to draw or write a description of what you hope life will look like again one day.

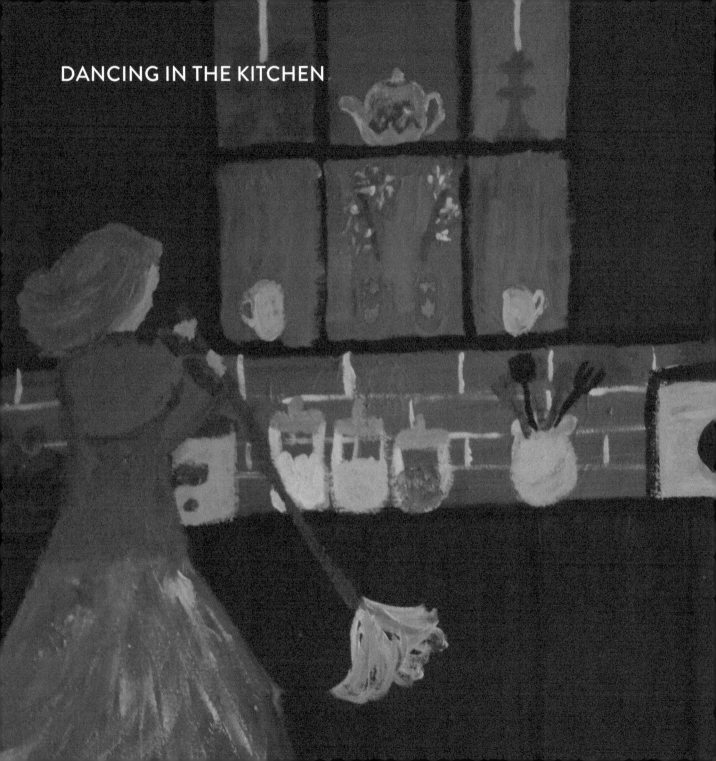

DANCING IN THE KITCHEN

31

Dancing in the Kitchen

You turned my wailing into dancing;
you removed my sackcloth and clothed me with joy.

(Psalm 30:11)

It was the summer of 2020 and I was talking to Chad Loftis, a counselor from The Well International in Chiang Mai, Thailand. I was telling him how I didn't want to end up bitter and angry. He said it was good that I knew what I didn't want to look like, but what did I want to look like?

Immediately, I thought of a story I read in a Patsy Clairmont book many years ago. The story was about a lady whose husband had left her. She was brokenhearted. Her adult children ached for their mother as she navigated the disappointment and learned how to manage life again. One day, much later down the road, her adult daughters walked into their mom's house to find her with her music on so loud that she didn't even hear them enter. As they searched for her, they found her dancing with the mop in her kitchen. What a picture of healing!

I answered his question, "Dancing in the kitchen."

That's my goal. That's who I want to be.

Although anger is a natural response to betrayal, if we allow it to lead us to seek revenge or bitterness, it becomes sin. That is not the direction God wants for us.

I painted this image to remind me of my goal.

I've worked hard on self-awareness and emotional health.

I'm taking medication for my anxiety and depression.
I'm trying to practice rest and stillness.
I am committed to reaching out when I want to hide.
I try to practice rhythms that will help me experience God's love.
I continue to receive counseling and to work on each layer of heartache that makes itself known.

I know the grief and trauma work I do now will help me in the future

I'm committed to this healing journey, even if it never results in restoration or a remarriage with my former husband.

But I hope it does result in dancing.

Lots of dancing!

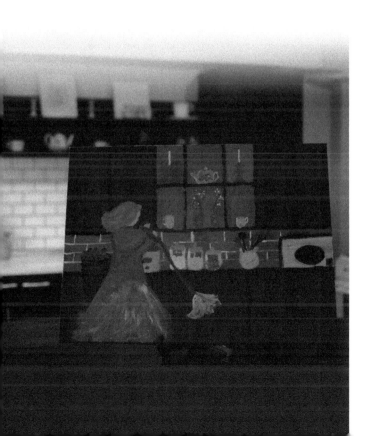

Questions *to* Consider:

1 Which rhythms in your life are helping you in your healing journey?

2 Take a look at the following. Are there any new actions or practices you would be interested in planning or starting today?

- making a daily list of griefs and gratitudes
- making an appointment with a psychiatrist to check your depression and/or anxiety levels.
- reading a Psalm daily
- checking in with a friend daily
- listening to a helpful podcast weekly
- making an appointment for a physical check-up
- scheduling physical exercise
- scheduling time for journaling, drawing, or painting
- listening to scripture as you fall asleep
- taking time for breath prayers throughout the day (for example, as you breathe in, you could pray "I need you" and as you breathe out you could pray "You are here."
- spending time in nature
- spending time with people who make you laugh
- others?

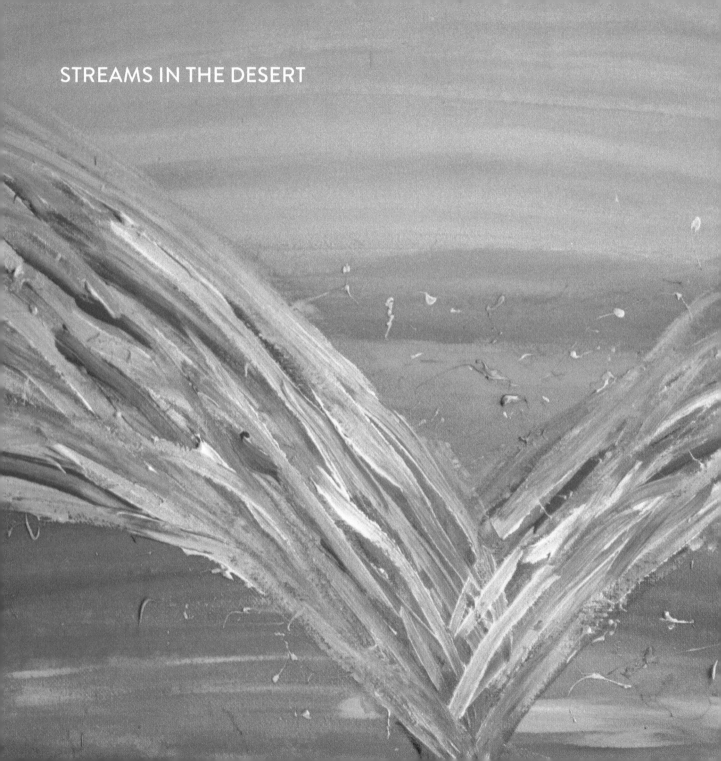

STREAMS IN THE DESERT

32

Life Giving
Community

"Behold, I am about to do something new; even now
it is coming. Do you not see it? Indeed, I will make a
way in the wilderness and streams in the desert"

(Isaiah 43:19 BSB)

"How are you, Sheila?"

My husband and I were facetiming with Greg and Stacey Oliver in the U.S.A. Greg and Stacey run an organization named *Awaken* where they help other couples going through sex addiction and betrayal trauma. They come from a story of their own brokenness and recovery, and I had heard them speak online and had reached out to them. We had been talking about my husband's story and his behaviors while they asked questions. After a while, Stacey stopped and seemed to look right at me through the screen and simply asked how I was doing.

I burst into tears. So much attention had been given to trying to understand and help my husband. I had not yet had time to process or look at my own pain. Her kindness and understanding poured life into my wounded soul. Hearing from someone else who had gone through the same pain I had gone through was deeply healing for me.

Over the years after D-Day, I would find many counselors, friends, mentors, and coaches who would help me along the way. Because of my spouse's blame-shifting, gaslighting, and manipulation, I needed validation that I was not crazy. I needed help unraveling the truth. I needed people who could speak truth and grace into my life. I needed to hear from people further along in the journey.

Between working on my marriage and feeling overwhelmed emotionally, I did not have the capacity to engage in all the familiar routines that had brought me community in the past. I had to cancel gatherings with friends. Sometimes I simply forgot appointments. I was anxious around groups of people. I'm sure my limited capacity most likely hurt some of my friends at that time because I was simply unable to participate in everything I had before.

I was hungry for podcasts, books and mentors who could give me language for what I was going through. I needed to hear stories of addicts who had found freedom. I needed to hear that wives had survived.

When we would travel to the states, I would set up meetings with those who I had heard online who had similar stories. I spent money to connect with betrayal trauma coaches. In Thailand, I often traveled to Chiang Mai to receive counseling.

I honestly don't know how I would have made it alone.

My husband's thinking, whether from mental health issues or sin, was distorted. I came out of every conversation feeling a cloud of confusion. One of the main ways that God ministered to my thirsty soul was by providing others who surrounded me with encouragement, prayer, and truth.

I was very fortunate to have people around me who believed me. As I have talked to other wives who have been told to not talk about these hard things, I have been very grateful for the godly friends, counselors and church leaders that God put in my life.

At times, the Enemy can accuse me of being so very weak that it has taken a multitude of people to help me survive these past few years.

But, I am not ashamed to admit that I have needed Truth-Tellers in my life.
I have needed to send a text in the middle of the night asking someone to pray.
I have needed each counseling session.
I have needed tear-filled talks and walks.
I have needed others to lift me up in prayer when I couldn't keep going on my own.
I have needed friends who act as cheerleaders.
I have needed trusted mentors to help me if I start to veer into bitterness or unfair judgement.
I have needed nourishing encouragement along the way.
I've needed laughter, which is truly medicine for the soul.

I've chosen to ask for help.

Each time, it takes vulnerability. And courage, too. It has resulted in seeing that there are friends who are willing to help. Although not everyone has had the time or capacity or understanding to help me, there have been some who have been willing to walk this hard journey with me. Some, just for a season. Some throughout the last six years.

I have heard Nate Larkin share on the Pirate Monk podcast that although each Christian has a personal relationship with God, it was never intended to be a private relationship with God.

God's design is for us to walk in community. That includes being willing to fight our pride or our shame in order to ask for help when we need others.

Without my community, I'm quite sure I would have perished in the desert. At the very least, I would have become a shell of who I am, with walls so thick around me that I couldn't truly engage with life again.

How thankful I am for the life-giving water of God's love displayed through community.

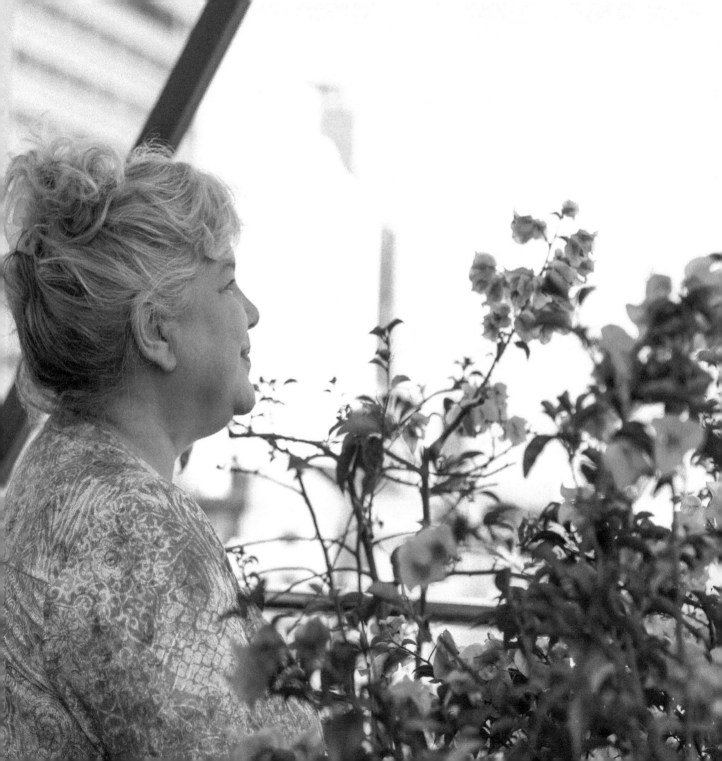

Questions *to* Consider:

1 Do you find it hard to ask for help when you need it? If so, why do you think it is hard for you?

2 Have you been able to pay attention to your own pain and needs during your trauma, or has all of your attention been towards the one who, for whatever reason, is in the center of the story?

3 How has your community been life-giving to you? If you haven't experienced this, yet, what might be some steps you could take towards establishing a supportive team around you?

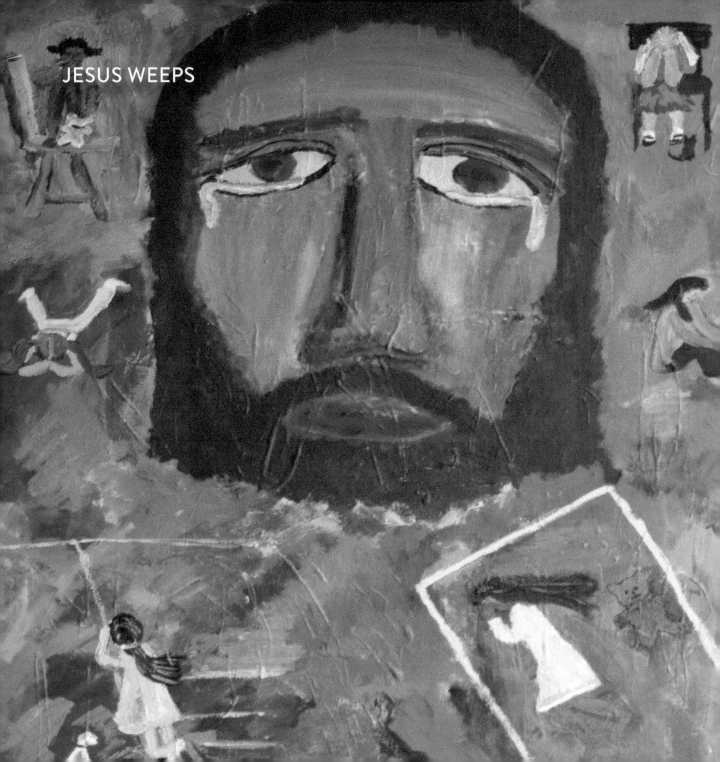

JESUS WEEPS

33

Little Girls
and Dreams

"The man who hates and divorces his wife,"
says the Lord, the God of Israel, "does violence to
the one he should protect," says the Lord Almighty.
So be on your guard, and do not be unfaithful."

Jesus wept. John 11:35

(Malachi 2:16)

My story is not the only one of a shattered heart.

Not too long ago, I was talking to a friend about her husband's porn addiction. As I thought back to our childhood, I could never have imagined that those two little girls would have ended up hurting in marriages with sexual brokenness issues.

I thought back to so many stories I have heard of abuse, rejection, and hurt that I have heard.

The first I remember was when I was thirteen years old. Another missionary kid shared with me (after swearing me to secrecy) that her father was coming into her room at night. A missionary, a man, a father who should be protecting his children was doing violence to the very precious one he should be protecting.

As I've worked with teens over the years, the deepest pain I have seen is when girls tell me about sexual abuse that has happened in their lives. Sometimes, it is the first time they can bring themselves to say the words.

So many girls' hearts are shattered.

And, I believe it shatters the heart of Jesus, as well. Just as He wept with Mary and Martha, I believe He weeps with us.

I don't know how many times I have been weeping, often laying on the floor in total agony. Only the picture of Jesus weeping alongside of me has brought me comfort.

I know He hates injustice.
I know He hates lies and betrayal.
I know He weeps when we weep over broken vows.
I know it hurts for Him to see what He has joined together now broken asunder because of secrets and unfaithfulness.
I cried as I painted this painting.
Crying for little girls who were not protected.

Crying for the grown women, like me, whose little-girl dreams had died.

One reason I fought so hard not only for my own healing, but my husband's as well, was because I want to see change in systems of thinking.
I want to see little girls and women believed when they have been treated unjustly.
I want to be a voice crying out for the protection of those who feel as if their voices have been silenced because of the injustices done to them.
I want to see Christian men rise up to examine their hearts and pay attention to the reasons they give in to temptation.
I want men to examine why they do what, on some levels, they don't want to do.
I want to see little girls protected at churches and schools and homes.
And if they are not protected, I want them to know where they can turn and what they can do to

get help. I want to see wives live in the light, and not in shame.

I want pretense and secrets to not have any place in the church.

I believe that the #metoo and #churchtoo movements have helped bring some acts of darkness into the light. May healing continue. May peace come to those hearts who have been violated.

Come, Lord Jesus, come.

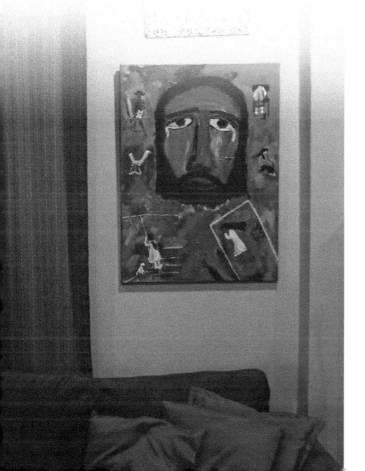

Questions *to* Consider:

1 What stories of mistreatment have you experienced or heard of that have to do with a misuse of a perceived power or authority?

- parents towards children?
- teachers/caretakers/adult relatives towards children?
- pastors/bosses/therapists/doctors towards members of the congregation, employees, clients, or patients?
- husbands towards wives?

2 Have you been the one to harm others, the one who has been harmed, a bystander, or someone who has traveled alongside someone who has been hurt?

3 Is God calling you to be an advocate for those who have been hurt?

4 How does the image of Jesus weeping with the wounded impact your heart?

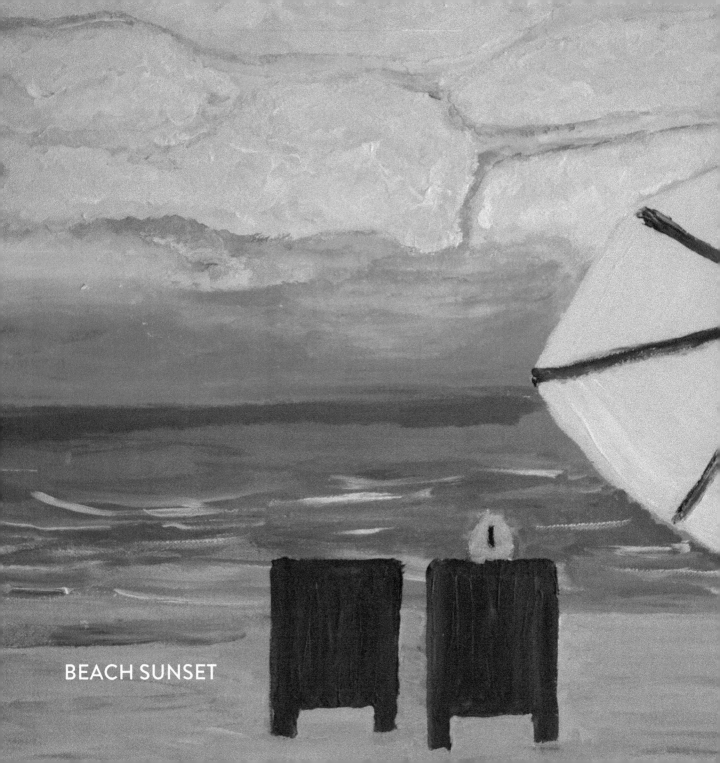

BEACH SUNSET

34

Romantic Moments

For your Maker is your husband— the LORD
Almighty is his name— the Holy One of Israel is your
Redeemer; he is called the God of all the earth.

(Isaiah 54:5)

I always loved romantic stories. As a child, I dreamed of meeting my prince. I could spend hours thinking about how it would happen. I could fantasize about sitting with my head on his shoulder. I could picture special picnics and dates. I could imagine candle lit dinners. I could see us standing at the beach, my hair and dress flowing in the wind.

As I'm sure you can tell, I loved fairy tales when I was little and romance novels as I grew older.

I started dating my future husband my freshman year in college. We dated throughout college and we were married our senior year. Many of my dreams came true...

... My first kiss on the bridge at the botanical gardens.
... Our sixth-month wedding anniversary at a romantic Bed and Breakfast Inn.
... Even after our home was filled with children, we were very intentional about date nights and overnights in romantic places. When we were low on money we would pretend to be in a fancy place or in another country while eating supper on our enclosed porch.

When I found myself suddenly single, I didn't know what to do with all my hopes and dreams that centered on romance. How could I ever go to the beach again? Would I ever light the candles in my house again? How could I enjoy dressing up and going out to a fancy restaurant?

When things started opening up in Thailand after the first wave of COVID, some friends (including my daughter and son-in-law) invited me to go to the beach. It was hard to decide what to do. I loved the ocean, but I dreaded going for the first time without a romantic partner. I knew I would have to face losses since many of our favorite times as a couple and as a family had taken place at the beach. I chose to go anyway.

One night, the others decided to go into town for dinner. I stayed at the resort and sat outside watching the sunset. Even though it was beautiful, I felt anxious. As I sat there, I felt God remind me that He was the Creator of all that I could see. Then I felt a question come to my heart.

"Sheila, can you just sit and enjoy my creation with me?"

I thought about this invitation.

Yes, yes, I could.

I could fully enjoy the moment knowing that God was sitting with me.

I was not alone.
I could enjoy my Maker's masterpiece and delight in His presence.

A setting that I had labeled as romantic could still be enjoyed in singleness.

Once when I was talking to my sister about romance and singleness, she laughed and said that when she was in a group of friends in high school who were not dating, they came up with the term "rotic."

Because romantic without the "man" is "rotic." That made me laugh!

She said they gave themselves permission to have rotic moments, even in their singleness! Because couples shouldn't get to have all the fun!

That's what I've decided to do, too.

So, I do strike matches and light the candles in my apartment.

I've dressed up to go to a fancy restaurant with a friend.

I've taken trips by myself to beautiful places.

I believe I have just begun on a journey of many more rotic moments in my future.

Questions *to* Consider:

1 Do you struggle with a narrative that your life cannot be enjoyed without a romantic partner? Or, maybe without something else...a certain place to live, success in your education, a specific job, etc?

2 What would it look like for you, in this moment of your life, to allow God to be enough for you?

3 Is there a step of faith you could take that would move you out of your comfort zone and more into the presence of God?

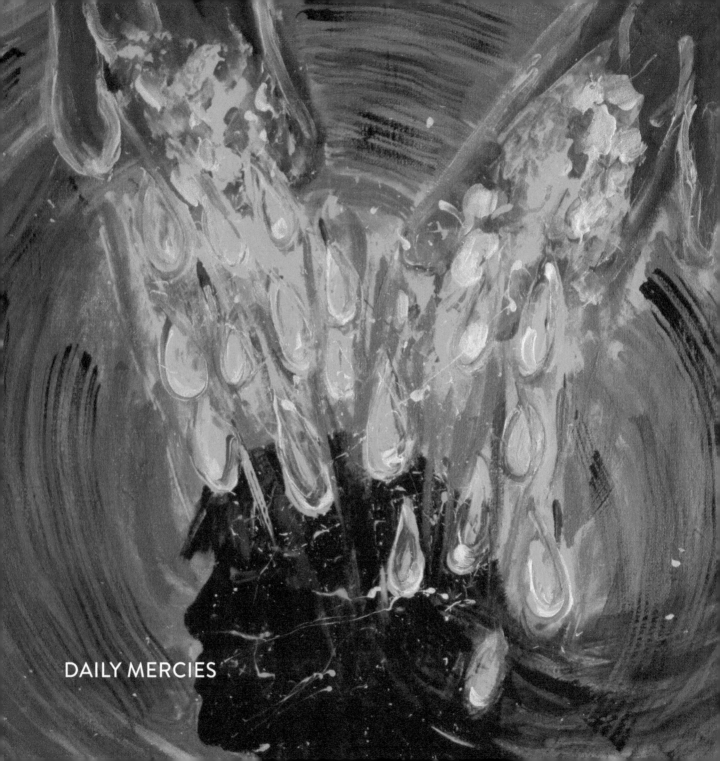

DAILY MERCIES

35

One Day at a Time

Because of the Lord's great love we are not consumed,
for his compassions never fail.
They are new every morning;
great is your faithfulness.
I say to myself, "The Lord is my portion;
therefore I will wait for him."

(Isaiah 54:5)

There have been so many times on this journey I have wanted to know what was around the corner.
Should we pay money for an intensive retreat?
Would my husband do the hard work of recovery?
Would our marriage survive?
Would things look better in a year?
If we were to move, would that make a difference?
Would the roller coaster ever even out?

God didn't reveal the future.
He just gave grace for each day.
One day at a time.

I remember one time when a member care counselor came to my place of work to meet with each employee. When she asked me how I was doing, I broke down. I cried and cried and shared with her the journey we had been on.

"It's like I've been so wounded that I'm lying on the floor. I keep telling myself to get up, but I can't. I have no energy and I can't think about anything else. I think my hope is gone."

"Just stay on the floor," she answered.

That surprised me.

"Yes, if that is where you are right now, then lie on the floor. Speak your grief and lament to the Lord. Let Him know you can't get up. One day, I bet you will be able to raise a bit on one elbow. Another day, I imagine you are going to be able to hold on to your sofa and pull yourself up to a sitting position. Eventually, you will stand and walk again. But don't try to force yourself to be somewhere you are not at."

That mental image stayed with me.

For a long time I couldn't make myself move forward.

Eventually, just as she said, I was able to make baby steps towards healing.

I painted *Daily Mercies* on a day when I couldn't seem to make myself do anything. I didn't really even want to paint and I had no clue what I wanted to paint. I swirled paints around on the canvas and just enjoyed the colors. Then the thought came to me that God's grace was like beautiful colors spilling on my head, and that it was enough for today.

It reminded me of the Israelites and the manna that God provided for each day. They couldn't store it because maggots invaded it and spoiled it. There was just enough for each day. What they needed for each day was provided.

God knows the portion we need.

One day at a time.

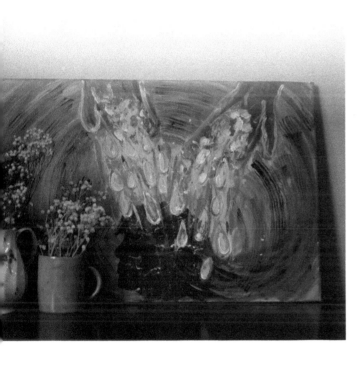

Questions *to* Consider:

1 Have you seen God's mercies in your journey or have you felt alone and abandoned? If you have seen God's mercy and provision, make a list of the ways you have seen Him at work.

2 Perhaps you feel alone, like you are lying in a heap and you can't get up. Hope may seem like a foreign word. Try speaking your grief and lament aloud to a friend or to your Creator.

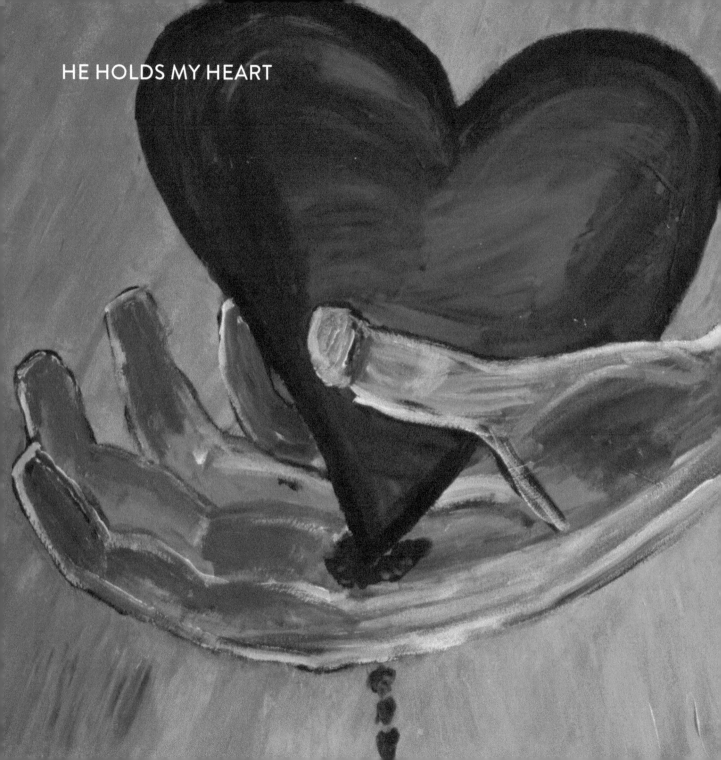

HE HOLDS MY HEART

The Price
of Love

But God demonstrates his own love for us in this:
While we were still sinners, Christ died for us.

(Romans 5:8)

I felt that love was going to kill me. I had given it freely and gladly to my husband and I had been terribly wounded from it. There were many days when I didn't know if I could keep going with the weight of the betrayal, the pain, and the grief.

It was the same with loving Kevin. His rebellion in his teen years and then his devastating suicide left my heart feeling pierced.
I had loved him for twenty-seven years.
I had believed in him.
In what he had to offer to the world. In the unique person God had made him to be.
Then, in one quick instant, he was gone from the world.

Yes, love hurts.

Somehow, through it all, I kept feeling that God was holding my heart.
That even though my heart felt ugly and lifeless, God was tenderly cradling it, breathing life back into me.
When I least expected it, there would be a supernatural sweetness I knew was the gift of God.

As I began to paint this image of God tenderly holding my heart, I realized that His love cost Him, too.
Love did kill Jesus because it was what prompted Him to come to earth and to die on the cross.
Choosing a close relationship with me had cost Him.

Because of my fragility and humanity, it was necessary that nails pierce the hands of Jesus. It was a deliberate choice God made because He loved each one of us.

Thinking about the cost of love was not the direction I had planned to go when I started the painting. But as I painted the hand of Jesus, it was as if He was crying out to me that there was a price to love and that I could not paint His hand without also painting the cost that came with it.

As C. S. Lewis said *"To love at all is to be vulnerable. Love anything and your heart will be wrung and possibly broken. If you want to make sure of keeping it intact you must give it to no one, not even an animal. Wrap it carefully round with hobbies and little luxuries; avoid all entanglements."*

I want a heart that continues to stay alive, even though cost will be involved.
I want to continue to love those that God has put in my life, even though there is always the risk of pain.
I know the beauty in love is greater than the pain.

I know that because I know that Jesus loves me.

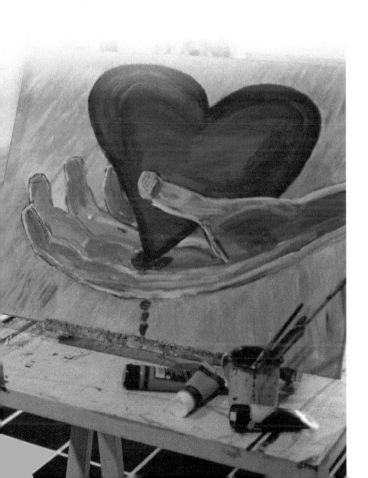

Questions *to* Consider:

1 How does the knowledge that Jesus was willing to love you, even though His love resulted in pain, make a difference in your heart?

2 What has been some of the costs of love that you have experienced with the love that you have given others?

3 If you have experienced a broken heart, have you been tempted to wall off your heart so that you won't experience any more pain? How has that worked for you?

4 Do you want to be able to love others well, even though it may require more costs from you in the future?

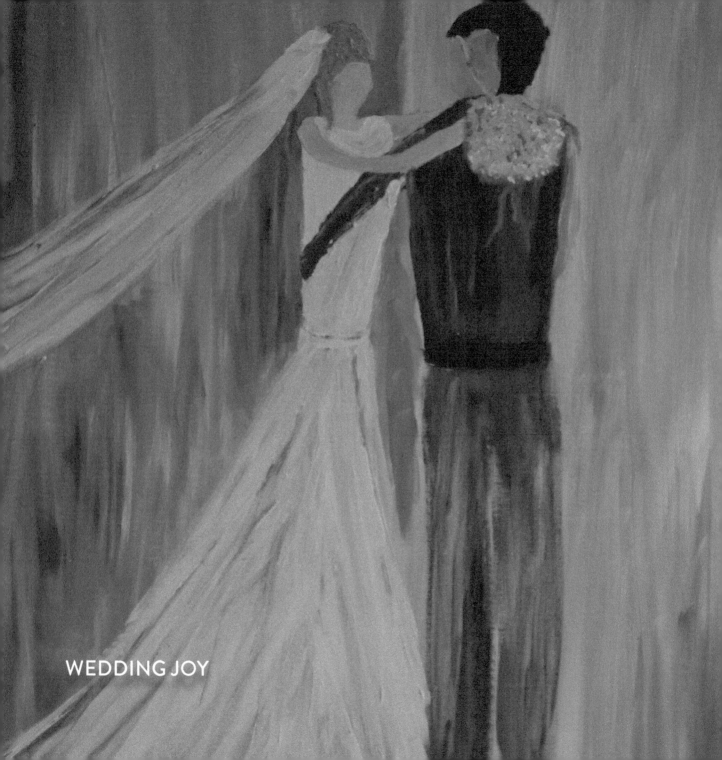

WEDDING JOY

37

View of Marriage

Christ loved the church and gave himself up for her to make her
holy, cleansing her by the washing with water through the word,
and to present her to himself as a radiant church, without stain
or wrinkle or any other blemish, but holy and blameless.

(Ephesians 5:25 & 26)

Let us rejoice and be glad and give him glory. For the
wedding of the Lamb has come and his bride has made herself
ready. Fine linen, bright and clean, was given her to wear."
(Fine linen stands for the righteous acts of God's holy people.)
Then the angel said to me, "Write this: Blessed are those who
are invited to the wedding supper of the Lamb!" And he added,
"These are the true words of God."

(Revelation 19:7-9)

I love a good wedding.

And I love the way God has given us the picture and reality of marriage as a foreshadowing of His great love for us.

I love that we get to look forward to participating at the greatest wedding celebration of all time!

One huge grief I wrestled with was the loss of my marriage. One day, I was on a phone call with a betrayal trauma coach. I was sobbing. I told her how badly I had wanted a marriage "til death do us part". I told her that, since I believe marriage is the most beautiful picture of God's love for us, I had wanted to show others what God's love looks like through marriage. I kept trying to get the words out between my tears of how much I valued marriage and how I didn't want to lose it.

She replied that I can still believe marriage is the most beautiful picture of God's love. It's just that one person can't hold a two-person commitment together. It doesn't take away my values and beliefs. I can still minister to others and share about the design God intended for marriage. The design of sacrifice and beauty. I can still love marriage.

That was so sweet to me.

When someone validated the pain of the loss of my marriage, that comforted me. It was good to know that others bore witness to the holiness and sacredness of marriage and the pain of watching it disintegrate.

Almost a year after the conversation with the betrayal trauma coach, my oldest daughter called to tell me she was engaged. I was grateful that I could rejoice and celebrate with her.
I could believe that her marriage could be what God intended it to be.
I could still believe that marriage is good.
I could still believe that God would equip His children for everything they need for such a huge commitment when they are each looking to Him and walking in obedience to Him.

I was able to anticipate and delight in the planning of my daughter's wedding, and when COVID restrictions thankfully lifted, I was able to go and be present at Joshua Tree in California when she got married!

The love of my daughter and her bridegroom was a beautiful reminder of God's love for me.

Questions *to* Consider:

1   How has your personal journey impacted your view of marriage?

2   Are you able to rejoice with others when they get engaged or married or have a wedding anniversary? Why or why not?

3   If this brings up tender emotions for you, take time to journal or to illustrate your emotions. Spend some time talking to God about how your views of marriage have been shaped.

4   Give God space and time to remind you of the Greatest Love Story-the story of His love for you.

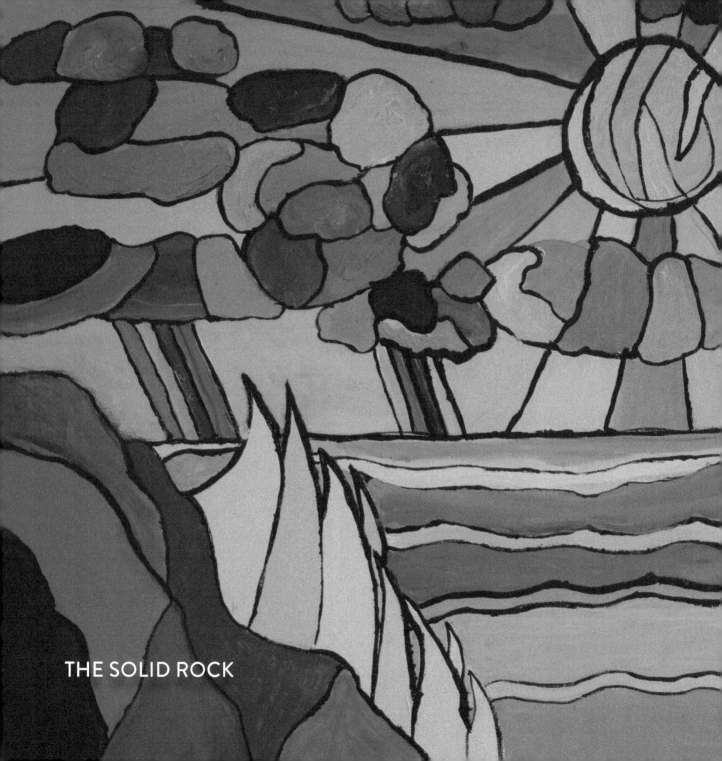

THE SOLID ROCK

38

A Firm Foundation

Jesus is the same yesterday, today and forever.

(Hebrews 13:8)

Therefore, since we are receiving a kingdom that
cannot be shaken, let us be thankful, and so worship
God acceptably with reverence and awe...

(Hebrews 12:28)

He lifted me out of the slimy pit, out of the
mud and mire; he set my feet on a rock and gave
me a firm place to stand.

(Psalm 40:2)

My heart was beating fast, not from the physical exertion of riding my bike to the school where I work but because of my anxiety. I was rounding up the school year during a pandemic, dreading the one year anniversary of my son's death, and wrestling with the fact that my husband had left me. I was a sleepless, grief-ridden mess. I had a long list of things I needed to accomplish as I finished my end-of-the-year checklist, cleaned my office, and put things away for the summer.

As I pulled my bicycle up next to the school, I saw my boss, the head of our school arrive, as well. I pushed my kickstand down as he greeted me. In response to his "good morning", I burst into tears.
As I cried, I somehow knocked my bike over. I took a step to pick it up and one of my shoes came off.
As we talked, my headmaster (and friend) quietly moved my bike.
Through my tears, I realized I had parked it right in the path people needed to walk to get into the school.
He kindly talked to me and then prayed for me as I tried to calm down.

Later, my daughter and son-in-law came by my office to cheer me along and to help me get everything done. I was grateful for the many ways God showed His kindness and provision to me even during the most difficult times.

This story of how unsettled and shaky I felt was one that could have been a comedy scene, if it hadn't been so sad.

So many days felt like sinking sand and I didn't know if there was anything firm beneath my feet.

My heartrate often accelerated, my hands often shook, my eyes began to twitch--there were certainly days when I didn't know if my heart and body would ever feel normal again.

During those shaky moments, I had to remind myself that I was part of a kingdom that could not be shaken.
I had to believe that God would lift me out of the slimy pit and that I would stand on a solid rock again.
I had to remember my confidence didn't come from circumstances but from God's promises.

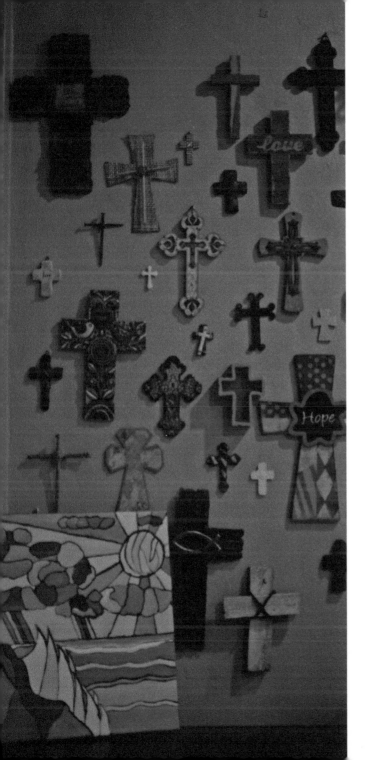

Questions *to* Consider:

1 Have you had moments in your journey where you have had panic attacks or when your anxiety was so high it seemed like everything was falling apart? If so, think about some of those moments.

2 How does the picture of a firm foundation in the midst of the storms and waves around you impact your heart?

3 Do you believe God can give you a firm place to stand...an unshakeable kingdom? Take some time to think about how this belief might influence your life.

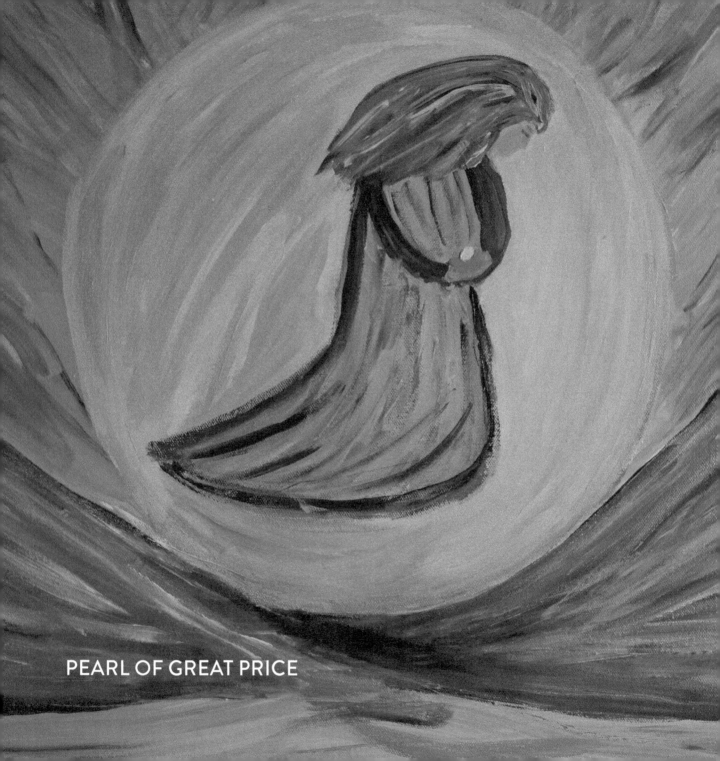

PEARL OF GREAT PRICE

39
Symbols

Again, the kingdom of heaven is like unto a
merchant man, seeking goodly pearls:

Who, when he had found one pearl of great price,
went and sold all that he had, and bought it.

(Matthew 13:45 & 46)

"Do not give dogs what is sacred; do not throw your
pearls to pigs. If you do, they may trample them under
their feet, and turn and tear you to pieces.

(Matthew 7:6)

On April 21, 1989 my best friend asked me to marry him. I answered "Of course!"

And he gave me a ring to symbolize his love. A few months later we were married and I was given a gold band to add to my ring finger. My rings weren't big or fancy but they were just right for me. How I enjoyed looking down and seeing that diamond sparkling up at me! For over thirty years, these rings had symbolized so much to me.

Being chosen.
Wanted.
Desired.
Loved.
Cherished.

The divorce date was getting closer and I didn't know what I was going to do about my rings. I felt like I couldn't take them off. How could I look down at a bare finger? Wouldn't it be crushing to have the symbols of love and hope stripped away?

Over the months as I worried about what I would do, I felt like God reminded me not to worry about the future because each day had enough worries of its own. Each time I felt the panic about the rings building, I would set that dilemma down to think about later.

When it got within three weeks of the day of the divorce, I could no longer set the worry down. I felt super anxious. I found myself having a tearful, emotional talk with God as I rambled on and on about my fears and frustration.

"It's almost here, Father, and I have no clue what to do. It's so painful. I don't think I can handle looking at a bare finger every day. It will feel so strange. But I can't wear these rings when I'm not married. They no longer mean what they once did. What will I do? These rings have spoken of love to me. How can I stand feeling a bare finger and looking down at it? It will be a symbol of rejection. What would you give me if you gave me a symbol of your love? How do you see me?"

"A pearl of great price." I heard the words in my soul immediately.

At first, I dismissed the idea that it was God speaking to me. I knew the parable about the pearl of great price. It was a story symbolizing the importance of God's kingdom and how valuable it is. It was not about me--a middle aged woman whose life was currently a mess.

I looked up information about the parable and was surprised to find that some scholars also believe the pearl of great price describes how God views His children. Allowing His son to die on the cross was how God gave up everything to keep the pearls of great price that He loves. I kept considering whether this image was from God.

A couple of nights later, while reading a fiction book, I was surprised to come across a description of the process of a pearl being formed in an oyster. It talked about how the beauty of the pearl originates when layer after layer is formed and placed over an irritant. Could it be possible that beauty was being formed in my life with each fresh hurt? Would a pearl be the symbol of the suffering I had endured and the promise of the beauty to come?

That same week as I was listening to the Bible, the verse about not throwing your pearls to the swine caught my attention. Pearls weren't meant to be placed where they would be trampled on, but where they would be treasured.

Again, I felt like God was telling me I was His pearl. He would value and treasure my life. He would not discard my heart and throw it away to be trampled on.

With great peace and joy, I went out and purchased a pearl ring. On the day that the divorce was finalized, I turned on a worship song. I sang it to the God who sees me as His beautiful pearl while tears dripped down my face. A deep sense of peace enveloped my heart as I exchanged my wedding rings for my new pearl ring.

Questions *to* Consider:

1 Have you felt like your heart has been trampled and torn to pieces? If so, how does the image of God valuing your heart and tenderly caring for it strike you?

2 How does the image of a pearl becoming more beautiful with each layer being formed over an irritant bring you hope for your future?

3 Can you picture God holding you, His pearl of great price?

4 What do you see when you look at this painting?

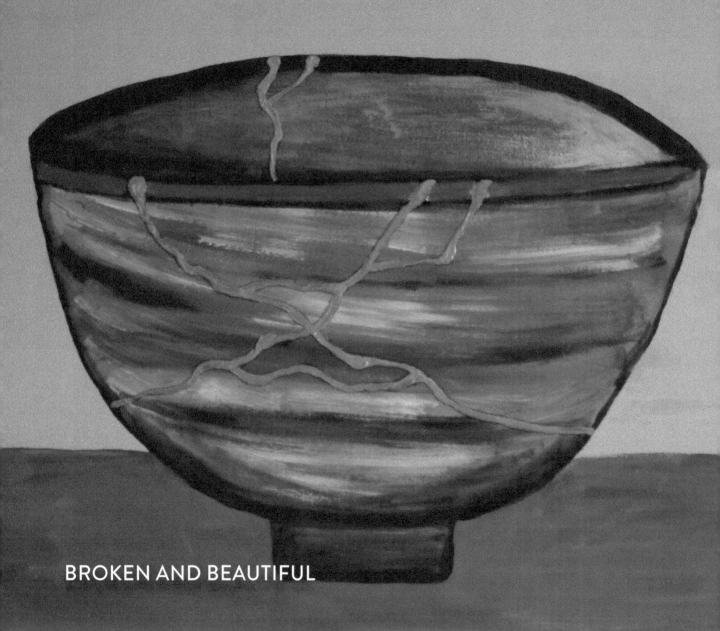

BROKEN AND BEAUTIFUL

Vulnerability

They triumphed over him by the blood of the
Lamb and by the word of their testimony.

(Revelation 12:11)

It's hard to open up and share when our stories are full of chaos and messiness. It's hard to expose our deep pain to others. For some reason, it seems much safer to keep our stories inside.

On the Pure Desire Podcast, I've heard Nick Stumbo mention often that sharing our stories is one more step towards our healing.

I did not want my pain to be wasted. If there is a chance that anything I can share will help other women on this journey, then I wanted to put a voice to some of my experiences.

When I first started painting, I meant it to be something just for me. I knew I had never had an art class and never excelled at anything artistic. I'd never even thought about it! But, after I began painting, I found it was a way I could show others my journey. At first I just shared my paintings with my family members and prayer warriors, but they encouraged me to share it with others.

In January 2021, I began an Instagram account. When other women wrote to me that a painting expressed exactly what they were feeling, it encouraged my heart.

It was affirming to know that something birthed in my pain was helping someone else.

One thing I have found that is not easy about vulnerability is the feeling of constantly having my needs and weaknesses revealed.

Often I feel too needy.
I feel I am constantly asking a friend to pray for me again, or listen to me express pain again.
It even feels vulnerable to ask for help in areas like finances or home upkeep—things that used to be taken care of by my husband but now have fallen to me.

After spending much of my life ministering to others, it has been hard to be willing to be the wounded one.

Perhaps it is easier to be a good Samaritan than to be the beaten and bloody one lying by the side of the road.

I have often heard that we can choose to push down the ugly and hard things, but eventually the pain from shame, grief and trauma will come to the surface. We can try to keep our shame submerged. Just like a beach ball held under water, the fallout from our trauma and shame will eventually pop up. If we don't talk about our sorrow, grief and guilt, those things will eventually come to the surface and be more damaging to our hearts and souls.

I'm learning the importance of being vulnerable and transparent, even when it is hard. I know that I want to be an emotionally-healthy person.

My job has given me many opportunities in regards to vulnerability. I learned years ago that when working with teenagers, it was extremely important to be authentic. They are not interested in adults who try to cover up real life with a picture perfect life. They want the real deal. In my job, I had always tried to be real with the students I work with. Even though it wasn't appropriate to tell them everything happening at home, I could share what I was learning about— whether it was brokenness, the gospel, shame, trauma, idols, and so many other truths. When it was time to let go of the marriage, I also had to find words to let them know that I was heading towards a divorce and that I was heartbroken because it was not how I wanted my story to go.

I think being in the position of leadership and being committed to transparency has been good for me. It hasn't been easy, but it has pushed me to put words to my story in appropriate ways.

I pray that trying to share my heart has pointed others to the only One who can heal our brokenness.

I pray that this is part of the triumphant story-- that what Satan meant for evil, God will use for good

Questions *to* Consider:

1 Kintsugi is the Japanese art where broken pottery is put together using gold—the flaws are highlighted to bring about an unusual beauty. As you think about your life, can you see any beauty that is developing (or has developed) from brokenness?

2 Have you thought about sharing your story in some way to encourage others… social media, sharing at a small group, writing a blog, etc?

3 Is there a way for you to share some of what God has been teaching you, even if you don't share all the details of the story?

4 As you contemplate sharing your story, does it sound like something you want to move towards, or do you find yourself pushing back against that idea? Invite God into whatever emotions you are experiencing.

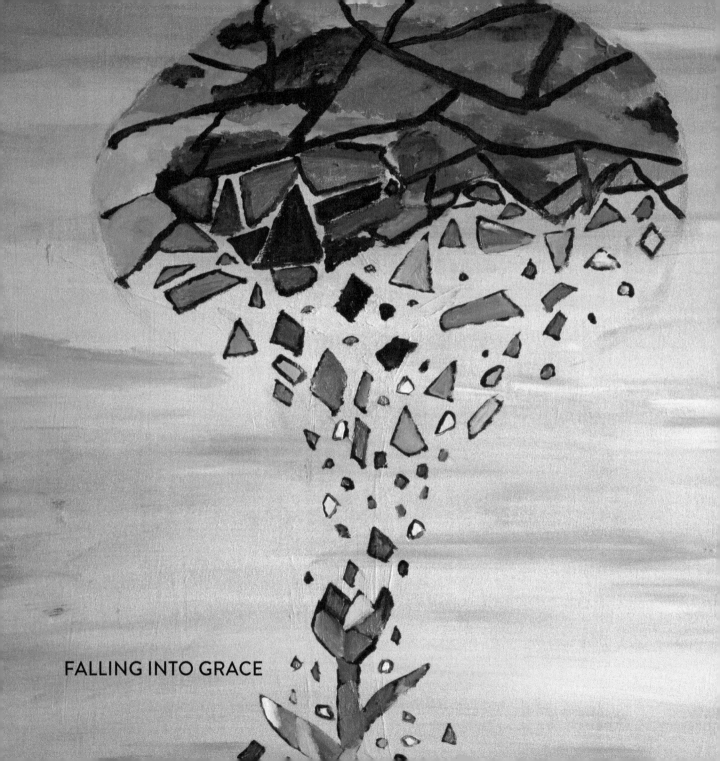

FALLING INTO GRACE

My World Fell Apart

Three times I pleaded with the Lord to take it away from me. But he said to me, "My grace is sufficient for you, for my power is made perfect in weakness." Therefore I will boast all the more gladly about my weaknesses, so that Christ's power may rest on me.

(Corinthians 12:8 & 9)

Immediately the boy's father exclaimed, "I do believe; help me overcome my unbelief!

(Mark 9:24)

It's not what I wanted.

I wanted to know that I was chosen and desired. Instead, my self-confidence was shaken and I felt unwanted and discarded.

I wanted to have a marriage that lasted until "death do us part."
To enjoy our grandchildren together.
I wanted to walk alongside my best friend into old age.
For one of us to tenderly take care of the other one when the ending of our life was beckoning, just like our parents had done.
I wanted our children to post pictures on social media of their gray-haired parents and remark "aren't they the cutest thing ever?"

But my world fell apart.
My dreams were in pieces.

My reality was totally different from what I thought it would be.

In some of my counseling sessions, I have been shown the illustration of the Sound Relationship House from the Gottman Method. The Gottman Institute website has more information about this theory. In this depiction, it is clear that the pillars of trust and commitment are needed to hold up the house. There is no need to work on the other important issues within a relationship (such as communication, finances, sex, etc) when the house is not standing.

Deception and ambivalence can kill a marriage, even when the other spouse wants to keep it breathing.

I'd watched the life I knew fall into a million pieces.

With each grief, loss, tear, fear, hurt, betrayal, minimization, justification, angry word and denial, another piece fell.

So now it comes down to belief.

Do I believe that God's grace is sufficient for me?
Do I believe His power will be made perfect in my weakness?
Do I believe that He brings beauty from ashes?
Do I believe that if I remain in Him, He will make my life fruitful again?

Sometimes I do.

Sometimes I have to pray, "I do believe; help me overcome my unbelief."

I hope something new and beautiful is growing out of the pieces.

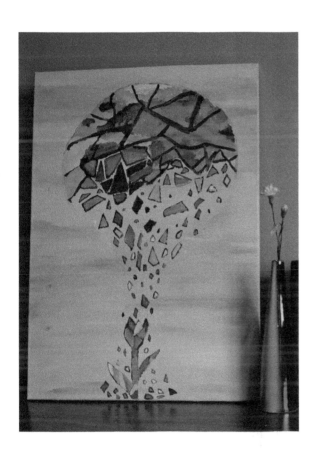

Questions *to* Consider:

1 As you look at this painting, how does it speak to you? Take time to journal about it or come up with your own illustration depicting new life coming from broken pieces.

2 Do you believe that your broken world can produce beauty? Why or why not? If you have a hard time believing this, spend some time praying the simple prayer, "I do believe, help me overcome my unbelief."

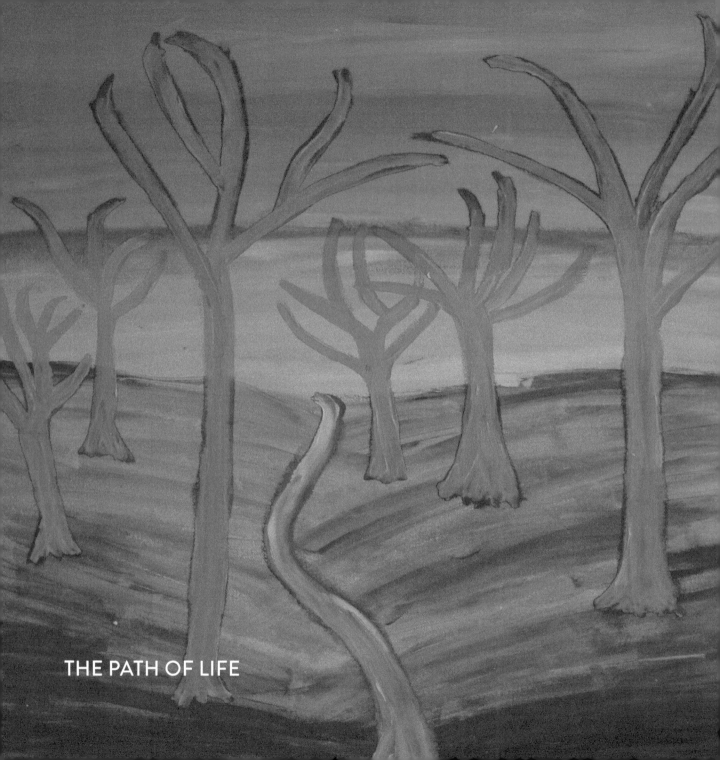

THE PATH OF LIFE

Into The
Unknown

The Lord himself goes before you and will be
with you; he will never leave you nor forsake you.
Do not be afraid; do not be discouraged.

(Deuteronomy 31:8)

You make known to me the path of life; you
will fill me with joy in your presence, with
eternal pleasures at your right hand.

(Psalm 16:11)

Even though I walk
through the darkest valley,
I will fear no evil,
for you are with me;|
your rod and your staff,
they comfort me.
(Psalm 23:4)

I'm glad I picked up that paintbrush on that day near the beginning of 2020. Painting has helped me grapple with my story. It's been a way to express myself when words have vanished. It's been a way to remind myself of God's promises, even in dark places.

Soon after my husband left, I knew I needed to do something about his office. I had to walk through it from my bedroom every time I went anywhere else in the apartment. As I looked at his familiar belongings, it made my home feel like a sad place. I was reminded that he had walked away from it all every time I stepped out of my bedroom. I was reminded that I was alone.

When I realized that painting was helping me to heal, I transformed his office into my studio. I filled the walls with bright paintings that spoke to me of my journey and God's faithfulness. It became a room filled with reminders of God's love for me through the valley of death. The death of a marriage and the death of my son.

I know I still have a lot of grief to process. I'm aware there will still be triggers ahead. There may yet be miles and miles to go on this healing journey.

I take one step at a time, trusting that God has a path for me...
Choosing to take Him at His word that He will never leave me nor forsake me...
Believing that He will not waste my pain...
Believing that because I am still breathing, there is still a purpose for me...

Anticipating the joy of His presence with every curve of the journey...

And, picking up a paintbrush when I need a reminder.

Questions *to* Consider:

1. As you think about the path that you are on, how would you describe it?

2. Are there any steps you could take today to remind you of the promises that are mentioned in the verses above—that God has gone before you, that He will never leave you nor forsake you, that He will make known your path to you, that His rod and staff are with you even in the darkest valley and that you do not need to fear what is coming ahead?

Maybe you can get an idea from this list:

- write out promises from God on sticky notes and place them where you will see them
- put a Bible verse as your screensaver
- purchase or paint a picture or verse and put it on your wall
- decorate a corner or a closet or even a room
- plant something new or put flowers in a vase
- use window paint or a white board marker to write on your mirror, your windows, or a sliding glass door
- set reminders on your phone to remind you to stop and pause to remember

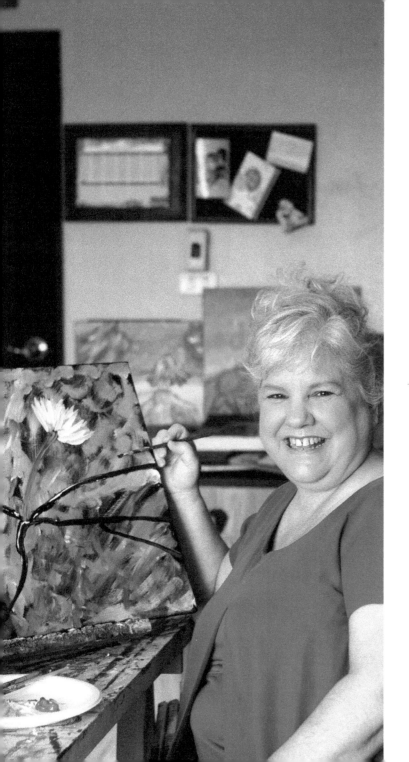

Acknowledgments

For as long as I can remember, my mother, Shirley Randall, has always asked me when I expect to write my book. Despite the fact that this was not the story either of us ever wanted, I am thankful that she has been my most faithful and enthusiastic cheerleader throughout this process.

My siblings, Mark Randall, Sharon Duvall and Susie Hansen, have also encouraged me all along on this journey. My friends Karen Groot, Suzie Person, Aimee Seaman, Staci Wolski, Lori Johnson and Brooke Cheser also spoke the right words time and time again to keep me going.

Many thanks to the photographers who worked with me—Tim Mills for his skills taking pictures of my paintings, and Verity Tan for the photo session of me in my studio. I'm thankful to have such talented friends! This was my first time to hire an editor, and I couldn't have been more pleased with the work of Yvonne Kanu. It was a pleasure to work with her—thanks, Yvonne! My designer, Shabbir Hussain, understood the importance of making this book visually appealing, and I am so grateful.

Many thanks to Nick Stumbo, Marsha Means, Jonathan Daugherty and Michael J. Cusick. Their ministries have helped me along this journey for the past few years and it was a special blessing to have their endorsements in my book!

I've saved my precious children for last, but certainly not because they are least! Even though I have tried to tell my personal story here, the events I share have been part of their story as well. As children who grew up in a secure home, the devastation of being hit with unclear thinking, hidden stories and divorce continue to leave them with a mountain load of grief and trauma to work through. How grateful I am that Maurissa, Shaina, and Isaac continue to turn to their Creator for grace and truth. How thankful I am that their spouses-Nate Edwards, William Gill, and Hattie Shea Harkins- provide loving and safe places for them. The births of Ezra Baer Harkins and Luna Ruth Harkins have brought the sparkle, delight and joy that we have needed! I've seen God's faithfulness not only to me but also to my children.

Grace upon grace. My heart overflows.

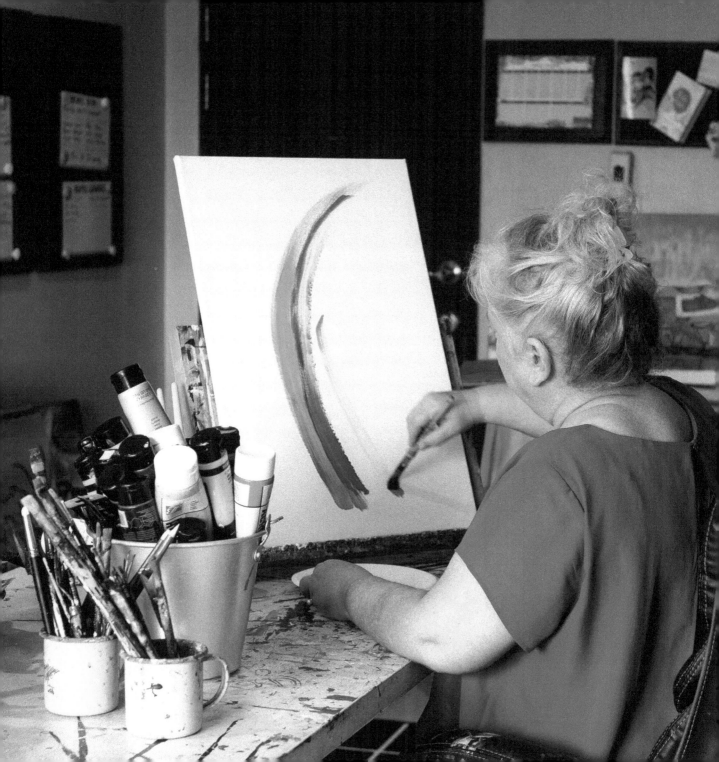

Sheila's Glossary

Addiction

A progressive brain condition in which the brain is negatively rewired due to a habit-forming substance or behavior. It includes preoccupation and continued use of the involvement even as the consequences rise. Because of the desire for the compulsive and pleasurable act or substance, the frequency of use, amount, and cost continue to rise. At some point, this leads to the individual being owned by the addiction rather than being able to control it.

Addiction Fog

This is the state that a person is in when their reward receptors are flooded with neurochemical dopamine. This creates imbalance in the limbic system of the brain and keeps the person looking for the next "rush" or "high" of experiencing the pleasure again. These gratifying sensations keep the addict from confronting any uncomfortable situations and keeps them seeking the next "fix." When in this state, the addict is not thinking clearly.

Acting out

These are outward behaviors of the inward fantasy life of a sex addict. These behaviors can include behaviors that society is generally accepting of and also those that violate the most significant boundaries our society has regarding sex. Therefore, acting-out behaviors can range from flirtation with someone other than their spouse, masturbation, pornography, hidden conversations and messages, exhibitionism, indecent phone calls, affairs, touching someone without their permission, and more severe and violent acts of sexual expression.

Ambivalence

The state of having mixed feelings or contradictory ideas about someone or something. In a marriage relationship, when the spouse who is acting out is ambivalent, they are not able to provide safety for the other spouse. The betrayed spouse is needing safety, but the ambivalent spouse is not sure if they can live within the boundaries of the relationship. Therefore, there is a constant roller coaster of "I want to, but I don't want to."

Betrayal Trauma

A type of trauma that refers to the pain and emotional distress when a breach of trust has occurred in a relationship you thought you could trust.

Blame-Shifting

When an addict does not take ownership of their behaviors and blames someone else. In a marriage with a spouse acting out, they often turn things around where the other spouse is blamed because of something they did or didn't do. It often includes the words "If you had" or "If you hadn't..."

Boundaries

A boundary is a limit to what a person is willing to accept from their partner. Examples can be as simple as "When you are late for a meal that I have prepared and the children and I are at the table and the food is hot, we will go ahead and eat instead of waiting for you to arrive." Or, as serious as "If you continue these acting-out behaviors and lying to me, I will have to pursue divorce."

Crazy Making

When an addict continues to live in denial, they often make accusations that make their partner feel crazy. The spouse then continues to question themselves and what actually happened. Facts are twisted and blame is shifted in a way that the spouse is constantly walking on eggshells around the addict and in a constant state of confusion.

D-Day

Discovery or Disclosure Day. It's the day the spouse finds out that there has been an act (or acts) of betrayal in the marriage. It reveals that there has been hiddenness, secrecy, and deception in the marriage. That day becomes the marker in the marriage of the before and after.

Delusions

A belief that is not based in reality. Both addiction and mental health issues can contribute to inaccurate beliefs.

Gaslighting

This is when one person convinces another one (through subtle words and behaviors) that what they perceive (their reality) is incorrect or inaccurate. I believe that this doesn't always come from a manipulative or harmful intention, but it can also come from a lack of self-awareness and delusional thinking.

Highs/ Hits/Rush/Euphoria: the intense pleasurable feeling that an addict feels when they have participated in the risky behavior of their choice.

Flooding

When trauma has occurred, emotional flooding can be triggered. The nervous system is on high alert. When triggered, the brain releases stress hormones that puts a person in flight or fight mode. Their heart rate and blood pressure rise. Breathing accelerates. As the adrenaline rushes in, a person in this state may not be at the best place for rationality.

Infidelity

At Affair Recovery, they define infidelity as the keeping of secrets. Although people often think of physical sexual affairs as the definition of infidelity, the actuality is that there are many ways for a spouse to be unfaithful to their partner. It can be from viewing porn, having hidden text messages, sexting, or going to sexual massages. I think it is safe to say that if there is cover-up in a marriage due to any emotional or sexual attractions and relationships, then there is infidelity.

Intimacy Anorexia/Intimacy Disorder/Intimacy Addiction/Approval Addiction/Love Addiction

There are many terms to describe motives or psychological reasons someone might be unfaithful in their marriage. Each situation is different and some of these terms may be more accurate than the more common "sex addiction" term that is usually the label given, especially if sex with another person is not involved.

Moral Suspension/Moral Justification/Cognitive Dissonance

The ability to redefine a behavior in order to have a reason to violate one's beliefs about right and wrong. The majority of people who act out even though it is against what they have stated they believe, do so after they find some "loophole" so that they can act out with little or no feelings of guilt.

Pornography Addiction

An addiction where the habit-forming behavior has to do with viewing explicit inappropriate content.

Post-Traumatic Stress Disorder (PTSD)

A mental health condition that gets triggered because of a traumatic event or series of events.

In betrayal trauma, the discoveries and revelations have rocked the safe world of the spouse. Various triggers result in anxiety, panic attacks, flashbacks, and other symptoms of trauma. Even though the discoveries may have happened months or years before, with PTSD you can suddenly feel as if you are back at the moment when your world was first shaken.

Psychosis

A more severe type of delusion where the person cannot distinguish between what is real and what is imagined.

Recovery

A return to a healthy state of mind. Both spouses in a relationship with infidelity will need to begin a recovery process. The addict will need to recover from his pattern of denial, acting out, and deception. The spouse will need to begin a recovery process as well. Even though they did not initiate the trauma, they will also need to enter a healing journey as their lives have been shattered. If they sit back and think that they are fine and don't face the grief, shame and trauma then they will most likely not heal.

Relapse

When an addict returns to the addictive substance or action after a period of sobriety.

Self-Soothe

Behaviors that are used to cope with anxiety, pain, or uncomfortable feelings. These can be helpful such as spending time with a pet or taking a walk. However, with addiction, these are often behaviors that are used to escape or to get a feeling like a rush or a "high", and they are harmful.

Sex Addiction

An addiction where the habit-forming behavior has to do with sexual fantasies or behaviors.

Shame

An isolating and paralyzing emotion that leads to self-doubt, feelings of unworthiness, and isolation.

Slip-Up

A behavioral lapse when a person returns to an acting-out behavior. It is different from a relapse in that the individual catches themselves, admits it to others and doesn't repeat it. Of course, if there are several slip-ups in a row, it then would be defined as a relapse.

Sobriety

In sex addiction, sobriety refers to the time that an addict has gone without the "acting out" behaviors they have decided are not healthy for them. Unfortunately, since fantasy is not able to be measured, an addict can look like he is sober, but he can be getting his "highs" from memories and fantasies. Just because someone has reached sobriety does not mean that emotional healing and recovery have taken place.

Social Shame/shared shame:

Addiction impacts family members in a number of ways. One of those is that they also experience shame, even though they are not the one struggling with the issue.

Trauma

Extremely intense and distressing situations.

Trickle Truth/Truth Dripping/Staggered disclosure

Facts gradually and reluctantly admitted by one's significant other especially about infidelity. This often takes place over a period of time, even though the addict insists each time that everything has been disclosed.

Triggers

Places, people, sounds, and smells that cause significant emotional distress because of a previous trauma.

Truth Tellers

People who you can trust to tell you the truth. This is the band of counselors and friends you will need to help you cut through the confusion of mental unhealth, gaslighting, manipulation, and blame-shifting. These are the people who take you back to grace and truth. These are people who you can send off a quick text to pray for you no matter the day or time.

White-Knuckling/white-knuckle sobriety

The state of ceasing acting-out behaviors by trying hard without admitting that the behaviors have become out-of-control. This is when an addict may stop behaviors to please others or with their own efforts. If they are white knuckling, they are not demonstrating the true change of recovery and they are not admitting that they need help.

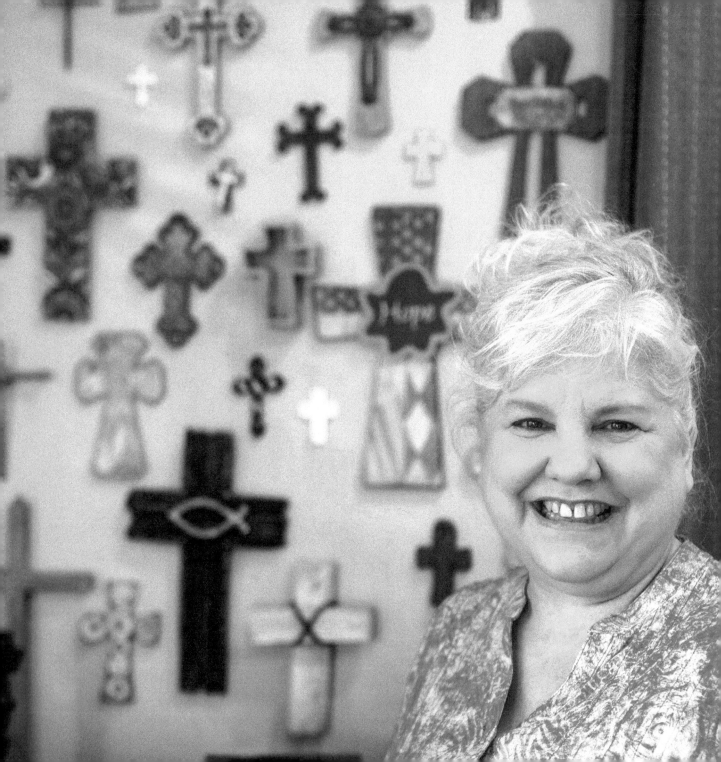

Suggested Resources

PODCASTS, VIDEOS AND WEBSITES:

A Circle of Joy website

Affair Recovery website and videos on YouTube

Awaken Recovery website

Authentic Intimacy website

Fight for Love podcast

Java With Juli podcast

Living Truth Podcast

Melody & Friends podcast

Pirate Monk Podcast

Samson Society and Sarah Society website and weekly group meetings.

Pure Desire Ministries website and podcast

Pure Sex Radio Podcast

Redemptive Living Radio

Restored 2 More Podcast

Restoring the Soul Podcast

BOOKS:

Shattered Vows: Hope and Healing for Women Who Have Been Sexually Betrayed by Debra Laaser

Intimate Deception by Dr. Sheri Keffer

Keep Walking: 40 Days to Hope and Freedom after Betrayal by Lynn Marie Cherry

From Betrayal Trauma to Healing & Joy: A Workbook for Partners of Sex Addicts by Marsha Means

Healing Your Marriage When Trust is Broken: Finding Forgiveness and Restoration by Cindy Beall

Worthy of Her Trust: What you Need to Do to Rebuild Sexual Integrity and Win Her Back by Jason Martinkus

Samson and the Pirate Monks: Calling Men to Authentic Brotherhood by Nate Larkin

Secrets: A true story of Addiction, Infidelity and Second Chances by Jonathan Daugherty

Healing the Wounds of Sexual Addiction by Mark Laaser

Going Deeper: How the Inner Child Impacts your Sexual Addiction by Eddie Capparucci

Surfing for God: Discovering the Divine Desire Beneath Sexual Struggle by Michael John Cusick

Addiction and Grace: Love and Spirituality in the Healing of Addictions by Gerald G. May

Unwanted: How Sexual Brokenness Reveals our Way to Healing by Jay Stringer

The Body Keeps the Score: Brain, Mind, and Body in the Healing of Trauma by Bessel Van Der Kolk

Rethinking Sexuality: God's Design and Why It Matters by Juli Slattery

Try Softer: A Fresh Approach to Move Us out of Anxiety, Stress, and Survival Mode--and into a Life of Connection and Joy by Aundi Kolber

WORKS CITED:

Chapter 4:

Keffer, Sheri. *Intimate Deception: Healing the wounds of Sexual Betrayal.* Revell, 2018. Chapter 20.

Chapter 6:

Slattery, Juli. Rethinking *Sexuality: God's Design and Why it Matters.* Chapter 2, E-book.

Chapter 8:

Beall, Cindy. *Healing Your Marriage When Trust Is Broken: Finding Forgiveness and Restoration.* Harvest House Publishers, 2011. Chapter 3, E-book.

Chapter 9:

Kolber, Aundi. *Try Softer: A Fresh Approach to Move us out of Anxiety, Stress, and Survival Mode – and Into a Life of Connection and Joy.* Tyndale Refresh, 2020.

Chapter 15:

Brown, Brene. "Shame vs. Guilt". Brene Brown. Accessed March 4, 2022. https://brenebrown. com/articles/2013/01/15/shame-v-guilt/

Aldis, Dorothy. *"I'm Hiding, I'm Hiding", A Child's First Book of Poems* by Cyndy Szekeres, Western Pub Co. 1981.

Chapter 16:

Reynolds, Rick. "Is Ambivilance Common When Healing From Infidelity? Accessed March 4, 2022. https://www.affairrecovery.com/newsletter/founder/healing-after-infidelity-paralysis-of-ambivalence-part-one

Chapter 17:

Means, Marsha. *From Betrayal Trauma to Healing & Joy: A Workbook for Partners of Sex Addicts.* A Circle of Joy Press, 4th Edition, 2020.

Chapter 23:

Daughtery, Jonathan. Secrets: *A True Story of Addiction, Infidelity and Second Chances.* New Growth Press, 2008.

Chapter 30:

Larkin, Nate. "It Starts with Attraction" Podcast with Kimberly Beam Holmes. Accessed March 4, 2022. https://www.listennotes.com/podcasts/it-starts-with/overcoming-sex-addiction-4TUBoR3f_tn/

Chapter 36:

Lewis, C.S. *The Four Loves.* B. Bles Publishers, 1960. Page 138.